Thriving Beyond Fifty

78 NATURAL STRATEGIES TO RESTORE YOUR MOBILITY, AVOID SURGERY & STAY OFF PAIN PILLS IN YOUR 50'S... AND BEYOND!

WILL HARLOW

ISBN: 9798642724736

DEDICATION

To Mum and Dad, who encouraged my reading and writing ever since I could hold a pencil.

To my grandparents, who are an endless source of inspiration (I hope you find something useful in these pages).

And to B, for showing me nothing but support, even during my early morning rituals.

"Don't let ageing get you down. It's too hard to get back up."

\- John Wagner

ALSO FROM WILL HARLOW

The 7 Steps to Overcome Sciatica - (2018)

TABLE OF CONTENTS

Introduction

First things first, I want to say "well done" to you for picking up this book!

By reaching for this book, then reading and applying the information within it, you'll be making a significant step towards improving your health - both in body and mind.

As the author of this book, my promise to you is that, even if you only apply *one* suggestion or piece of advice from the following pages, you'll find noticeable health benefits that will put you in better stead for facing the next ten, twenty or thirty years ahead. While this book was not written as a solution for any specific health problem or to provide you with a diagnosis, the information within it can help you to stay healthy, happy and avoid the most common problems I see people suffer with each and every day.

If we don't know one another, I am the clinic owner and lead physiotherapist at my practice in Surrey, UK, called HT Physio. I set up my practice to help people over fifty years of age to overcome painful problems, avoid unnecessary surgeries and get back to living their active lives. You can read more about my practice and what I do by visiting **https://ht-physio.co.uk**.

I wrote this book for people who know there is still so much living to do after the fifty year mark. I like to think of fifty as the halfway point in life; living to a hundred years old may seem farfetched, but getting there is becoming more and more realistic with each passing decade. The problem, though, is this: many people live to a wonderful age, yet suffer from nagging painful problems for these latter years. This can turn the final decades of your life from being potentially the most rewarding, to the most cruel and painful. Where I believe you should be exploring the world and enjoying time with your grandchildren after retirement, many people end up slowing down, forced into a sedentary life through poor health.

In my eyes, living with daily pain is no way to live at all and certainly shouldn't be seen as inevitable as we get older.

Of course, I'm not suggesting that it's possible to grow old without suffering any pain whatsoever; our biology is working against us in some respects. However, a large number of the problems I see every day and help people recover from are actually preventable!

The sad truth is that many people I meet have suffered for far too long with their painful problem, simply because they accepted that this is the way it has to be. If I achieve nothing else with this book than encourage you to believe it's possible to improve the outlook of any long-standing painful problem you may be currently experiencing, then I will certainly be content!

An additional aim I want to achieve with this book is to challenge the way we think about what our bodies can do as we get older. We automatically assume that a 25-year-old should be able to lift a suitcase or pick up a small child, but why do we accept the fact that only a handful of 80-year-olds can do the same? Of course, there's no denying the fact that muscles atrophy and lose their strength as we age, and some of our joints will inevitably show signs of wear to the cartilage, but these problems alone don't automatically determine whether or not we will be capable of performing physical tasks when we're older. In my opinion, we *can* strive to stay fit, healthy and strong as we get to 80-years-old and beyond... but we *must* start now. This is backed by a growing body of research that swells year on year.

In the first section of this book, I discuss the fundamentals of strength, mobility and ageing, and show you how to challenge the "inevitable" process of age-related deterioration that occurs in many... but not in all. My encouragement is for you to strive to be in that smaller group, the group that defies the ageing process, remaining fit and capable through their advancing years, despite the so-called odds being stacked against them.

How to Read This Book

If you're like me and you believe we should take care of our health as if it's our most valuable asset, then I know you'll enjoy the content of this book and will find the information useful. Because health is such a wide-ranging topic, I've written this book in a way that will be digestible for the reader who wishes to read it straight through, cover to cover. I have split the book into a number of sections - separating the body into its respective parts and the mind into a separate section - to help you navigate your way through the pages and pick the parts of the book that are most relevant to you if you so wish. If you wish to flick from section to section, I would strongly recommend keeping a finger on the table of contents, using this as a reference point if you prefer to just read the parts relevant to you. I would, however, suggest reading this book in its entirety if you have the time (provided you find my writing engaging enough to hold your attention, of course). You may find some nuggets of wisdom and information you can apply to your life right away, even in the chapters that you didn't expect to be applicable to you.

Within each chapter of the book, I've attempted to unpick the reasons behind, as well as the solutions for, a number of the most common health problems people face that are either preventable or treatable. You'll learn how to prevent and treat more than one type of shoulder pain. You'll read how arthritis might not necessarily be inevitable and how all hope is not lost if you've got the early signs already. You'll learn how not to fall (and so give yourself the best possible chance of avoiding lengthy hospital stays). I'll even show you some compelling evidence for techniques to mitigate the risk of dementia and depression, a feat once thought impossible.

I've attempted to back up all the information provided with scientific evidence wherever possible; you will find a reference list at the end of this book if you wish to peruse further or check my facts. I also wanted to include a free, yet incredibly valuable resource to the readers of this book. You can learn more about what that is and how to get it when you reach page 220 (or, if you simply cannot wait, flick to the last page and find out what it is now!)

The first of my two requests from you, dear reader, is that you approach the information in these pages with an open mind. You may read some things that surprise you, or that challenge the beliefs you currently hold. That is absolutely OK - I'm not asking you to change your opinions or blindly believe my writing, just that you weigh up the evidence and the information I present and make up your own mind. My second request is that, if the information I present in this book sits well with you and you've got the "all clear" from your doctor, you apply it to your own life.

Before applying any of the information in this book, it is important that you seek advice from your doctor. As it is unlikely that we know each other, you must always get approval from your doctor before implementing anything you read in this book. There is a clearly labelled disclaimer in the following section which I advise you read before continuing with the book.

Your health is your greatest asset. We only get one chance at living a long, healthy, comfortable life. My objective with this book is to give you some tools to improve yours.

Important Information

Throughout this book, you'll read information, strategies, techniques and exercises (henceforth referred to as "strategies") I've used with my clients to help them improve certain aspects of their health or fitness. These strategies should not be taken as medical advice, and should never be used as a substitute for individual medical advice from your doctor or the healthcare professionals involved in your care.

You shouldn't put into action any of the strategies from this book without first consulting your doctor about whether the strategies are suitable for your personal circumstances or not. Therefore, please do check with your doctor before you put any of the strategies into action.

If you do choose to follow any of the strategies in this book, you do so at your own risk. While I have made every effort to ensure the strategies I recommend are extremely safe, there will always be people that will not benefit from certain strategies in this book. Therefore, use your own sense and judgment when deciding whether the strategies in this book are suitable for you.

Making changes to your health or exercise regime carries risks, including, but not limited to, worsening of your condition, sustaining injury or failing to achieve the results you set out to achieve. Therefore, please weigh up all pros and cons with your own doctor before putting any strategies into action.

Please be aware that no strategy is 100% successful with everyone. I cannot guarantee your success if you choose to follow the strategies within this book. Please also be aware that there exists no provider-patient relationship established between the reader and the author as you work through this book. Never disregard any advice from your doctor or healthcare professional because of something you read in this book.

CHAPTER ONE

Cracking the Fundamentals

Before we dive into this book, I want to provide you with a short summary of some of the common terms I use in this book. I've tried not to let the *"curse of knowledge"* from my years of practice as a physiotherapist make my writing confusing. However, if you come across a term or phrase that you are unsure about, please rest assured that is my fault and not yours! Where possible, I have tried to explain terms and phrases as we go through the book, but this section may help you further. Think of it as a point of reference if you ever find yourself unclear.

- **Bone**: The strong structures that make up your skeleton, made of collagen (a protein that provides a soft framework) and calcium (a mineral that hardens and strengthens the bone).
- **Muscle**: The fleshy parts of our body that contract to produce movement. Muscles contract, and when they contract they pull on a bony attachment. This pulls one bone towards another, thus producing movement. Muscles cannot "push", only pull.
- **Tendon**: A tendon is the structure that joins a muscle to a bone. While these structures might look like a simple piece of string or rope to

the untrained eye, they are very complex (which is why they often cause problems).

• **Ligament**: A ligament is a fibrous band that joins bone to bone. Ligaments are strong bands of collagen and are much simpler in their composition compared to a tendon. You can think of ligaments as the parcel tape that keeps a cardboard box in shape. We have ligaments securing every joint in our body.

• **Joint**: An area where a bone meets another bone. A joint is formed when ligaments attach two bones together and the two (or more) bones articulate with one another. Joints allow movement; muscles either side of the joint pull on a bone to produce motion. We have a variety of different joints in our body, including hinge joints (like the knee) and ball-and-socket joints (like the shoulder).

• **Spine**: The bony part of your back and neck. We have 24 moveable bones in our spines (called vertebrae) plus a sacrum and a coccyx (the two bones that make up your bottom and "tail" area).

• **Core**: When we mention the term "core", what we are referring to is the muscle group that acts like a corset to keep our midriff stable when we walk, sit and move. Without a core, you'd be a floppy disaster. We all have a core, but strength between the core of two people might vary greatly (usually due to training, or lack thereof).

• **Cervical**: In the context of this book, the term cervical means "to do with the neck". You have 7 bones in your neck, called the cervical vertebrae.

• **Thoracic**: This term refers to your mid-back. You have 12 thoracic vertebrae.

- **Lumbar**: This refers to your lower back. In your lumbar region, you have 5 vertebrae. They are the biggest vertebrae in the spine.
- **Disc**: This refers to the intervertebral discs that sit between each and every vertebrae in the spine. They are comprised of an outer sac that holds a jelly-like liquid in the interior. A disc prolapse is a type of injury where the jelly-like substance pushes out of the disc and can irritate a nerve.
- **Muscle imbalance:** We always have more than one muscle at work around any one given joint in the body. Usually, muscles work as a team; one muscle might stabilise the joint, while the other contracts to produce movement. However, this process can sometimes go wrong and cause a problem with motion, often leading to pain. This is referred to as a "muscle imbalance". They can often go unnoticed for many years before seemingly "suddenly" leading to a painful problem.
- **Cartilage**: The cushioning and lubricating material that sits within every joint, between our bones. Cartilage allows normal, pain-free movement of our joints.
- **Arthritis**: Arthritis, or osteoarthritis, is a process characterised by the loss of cartilage in a joint, thickening of the bone, the formation of tiny cysts in the bones, and basically just general deterioration of a moveable joint in the body. Despite common belief, pain from arthritis is NOT an inevitable part of ageing. Many people have arthritis and experience no pain whatsoever.
- **Nerve**: The structures that carry messages from our brain to our muscles, telling them to move after our brains initiate the message. Nerves also transmit the signals that cause us to experience pain.

• **Inflammation**: A natural process that occurs within the human body whereby certain chemicals are released by the blood vessels that cause swelling and often pain. Inflammation isn't always bad; it is a natural response to injury and adaptation.

• **Mobility**: Discussed in two contexts; firstly, mobility can refer to how well you can generally get about on your feet, or up and down from a chair. This can be called "general mobility". Secondly, mobility can refer to the movement capacity and control of a specific joint. This can be called "movement-specific mobility". Think of the term "mobility" in both senses to describe how well one can move.

• **Flexibility**: Has a subtle difference to mobility in that it describes how much movement there is in a joint, regardless of control. I meet some young patients who have tremendous flexibility (they can bend forward and put their hands flat on the floor) but terrible control. They, therefore, have good flexibility but poor mobility.

• **Strength**: The ability to generate force using the muscles. In general, having greater strength is almost always a positive thing. This is why I speak about the importance of getting strong many times in this book (flip to the final page in this book for a free gift to help you with this goal).

• **General activity**: The amount of movement you carry out in any given day as part of your normal, daily routine.

• **Exercise**: Any activity you carry out with the express goal of getting fitter, stronger or more mobile.

- **Endurance**: The "staying power" you have in your heart, lungs and muscles during physical exercise. The better your endurance, the longer you can go on.
- **Resistance training**: A type of exercise with the goal of strengthening a group of muscles in the body. This could include weight lifting or body-weight exercises, like push ups.
- **Cardiovascular training**: A type of exercise with the goal of improving endurance as well as lung and heart health. Cardiovascular training doesn't make your muscles strong, but it does make your heart strong, and you fitter as a result.
- **Mobility training**: A type of exercise with the goal of improving the capacity for movement and control around a joint or area of the body. This does include certain types of stretching exercises, but gaining control of these new ranges of motion is the most important part of mobility exercise.

The Process of Ageing

All plants and animals age with each passing year. Unfortunately, we humans are no different. While we all have a good idea what ageing looks like for many people, why do these physical changes occur? And why do some people look far older than others, despite being the same age?

The visible and internal effects of ageing occur due to the process that the cells in our body undergo with each passing year. The cells in our body multiply to replace old cells at different rates; some replicate very frequently (like skin cells) while others are hardly replaced at all (like brain cells). Each cell has a finite number of times that it can replicate to produce a brand new cell. Once it reaches this limit, the cell dies and is re-absorbed by the body. As these cells are lost or damaged, the process of ageing starts to show.

Our skin starts to become thinner and show wrinkles as a result of a steady loss of skin cells. The surface of our skin becomes visibly drier as we produce less sweat and oil as we age. Under the skin, our bones become more pronounced under the skin as we store less fat in these visible areas. The rate of bone loss accelerates to outweigh the rate of bone growth occurring in our bodies. Our muscles lose mass and strength, meaning we can't run, jump or lift as easily as we once could.

But it's not all doom and gloom! With age comes wisdom, different perspectives and a wealth of experience, unmatched by the youth of today. What's more is that some of the processes of ageing aren't just negotiable - they are actually reversible. With effort and the right regime, it is possible for older individuals to reverse the rate of muscle loss within their body and actually become stronger. I have seen it with my own eyes on many occasions. The first and biggest step is accepting that it is possible and that a slow, ageing decline is not inevitable.

One of the reasons ageing happens seemingly so quickly for many is that they succumb to the temptation to make life easier by design as they grow older. Gradually decreasing their activity levels with each passing year, as family members constantly remind them to "take it easy", they lose vital steps each day. If you choose to become more sedentary over time, you'll gradually lose the ability to carry out the key fundamental human movements (explained in a few pages' time) without even realising it. Once you lose the ability to perform these fundamental movements, there will likely be situations where you'll need the assistance of others. You'll live with a higher risk of injury and your mobility and independence could even be threatened in advancing years.

I don't wish this loss of mobility and independence on anyone. This is why I've laid out the movements I believe to be key for over-50's (The Nine at Ninety) to protect and maintain vitality as the years advance. With some awareness, persistence and discipline, it's possible to practice and regain these movements should you find that you struggle to perform them as well as you'd like. You can find these fundamental movements on page 26.

The other part of us that can be affected by ageing is the brain. It is a common misconception that problems like dementia and Alzheimer's Disease (AD) are directly caused by the ageing process. Dementia and AD are *not normal* human processes and we shouldn't just expect and accept that they are a fact of life. In this book, we'll talk about strategies for keeping the brain, and the mind it contains, young and nimble.

Research carried out over the last fifty years has unearthed the fact that our fate is not entirely dictated by a pre-determined destiny. Major causes of death and disability, such as AD, that were once considered part of the genetic lottery, have been exposed as, to some extent, a result of the way we live our lives. This growing body of research is monumentally exciting; it puts our destinies back into our hands. For example, one of the key mitigating factors against AD isn't a pill or medication, but exercise. We will talk about the positive effects of exercise, which are simply too compelling to ignore, in this book more than once.

So, while ageing was once regarded as simply the inevitable process of moving closer and closer to the grave, we can now view it in a different, modern, more informed and hopeful way. It is important to realise that we have a choice as to how we live through the ageing process. We truly can control ageing when it comes to our health, fitness and mobility, and the ageing process of our brains is largely within our control too. This mindset may be one of the most important shifts you'll need to make to get the most out of this book.

Once you have internalised the fact that you do have a choice when it comes to how growing old feels, looks and plays out for you, you'll feel empowered to start making positive changes. And maybe you'll stop rolling your eyes and saying *"I guess I'm just getting old,"* whenever you get a new ache or pain!

What Is Mobility?

Mobility is the term given to two different aspects of your physical health. One definition of mobility is simply how well you can move about. Having good mobility means you can get out of a low chair, climb stairs and even adjust your feet quickly to react to a trip more easily than someone with poor mobility.

The second definition of mobility is body area-specific. This type of mobility refers to how well we can control the movement of a particular joint throughout it's complete range of motion. For example, you may be able to raise your arms over your head, but how stable are you when you get there? Do you have enough control to perform an intricate task, like changing a lightbulb? Having control throughout a range of motion is one of the most important parts of injury prevention and something we talk about a lot throughout the course of this book.

Both types of mobility are crucial to leading a long, happy, healthy life. Of course, they both feed into one another. Maintaining the ability to get about is only possible when you have good control through the joints in your lower limbs. Maintaining this good range of motion is only possible when you remain active and regularly use the movement capabilities available to you. We're going to call the first type of mobility "*general mobility*" - the ability to get about easily. We're going to call the second type of mobility "*movement-specific mobility*" - the ability to control the movement of a specific part of your body.

How do you know whether you have good general mobility?

The answer to this question really lies in what you'd like to be able to do in terms of movement each day. Good mobility for someone who works an active job and likes to take long walks on the weekend might look different than good mobility for an 86-year-old who just wants to be able to collect their paper from the shop every morning.

If you want to assess or improve your mobility, the first thing you should do is to write down what you'd like to be able to achieve each day without pain, feeling tired or feeling the need to stop when you're out and about. For example, you might decide that you want to be able to take the dog out for a 20-minute walk each morning, get into the gym three times each week and be able to go for one 2-hour walk every weekend without having to crash on Sunday because you're so worn out. Start by writing down the activities you'd like to be able to achieve each week. Be specific with distance and duration.

Once you have your list, I want you to write down what you're currently doing each week in terms of general activity. Look at the two lists and compare. You may currently be doing 70% of what you'd like to be able to do. This is fine; simply make a resolution for yourself, starting right now, that each week you're going to add 5% to your total activity level, until you reach your general mobility goal.

You may already be at 100% of your goal general mobility level. This is also fine; make a resolution to continue with this level of general mobility, and when you feel it slipping, you'll know to take action early as opposed to being oblivious to your mobility levels as they slip away. As you'll now be more aware of your activity levels, you'll be able to tot up a total of your weekly activity and compare it to your goals. If you miss a dog walk one morning, you'll know you're only at 95% for your general mobility quota that week, so you might add another 20-minutes onto your long walk on the weekend. There are endless ways to make up the general mobility quota you set for yourself; it just takes a little planning and preparation to do so.

How do you know whether you have good movement-specific mobility?

It's possible to assess the movement-specific mobility of every single joint in the body, and this is something I do regularly with my clients in my clinic. However, for the purpose of this section of the book, we will focus on testing your shoulder, hip, knee and ankle mobility. If you feel that you lack mobility in these or in other areas of the body, you will be able to find some guidance on how to improve these sticky areas elsewhere in this book.

- For the shoulder, you should be able to lift your arms high above your head without pain and without arching your back. You should also be able to reach up behind your back as far as your shoulder blade, as if to reach for a bra strap. Going in the other direction, you should be able to touch the back of your head with ease while letting your elbow roll out. If any of these movements are tricky for you, you may lack shoulder mobility.

- For the hip, you should have no trouble putting your shoes and socks on. Getting in and out of a car should be easy without having to turn your body and "reverse" back into the seat. If you have difficulty getting in and out of cars (especially low ones), or need to use a shoe horn to put on your shoes, your hip mobility may be poor. A bit of effort to improve it would help to safeguard this area of your body from future problems.

• For your knees, you should be able to squat down and pick something up from the floor by bending your knees, without having to rely on bending at the waist. When sat on a sofa with your legs up on the seat stretched out in front of you, you should be able to lock your knees out so that they are fully straight. If there's a slight bend in the knee when you do try to lock the knee out, you may lack full extension of the knee joint. This can lead to problems with walking.

• Finally, for your ankles, you should be able to squat so your thighs are parallel to the floor without your heels lifting up from the ground. If you can't do this because your ankles or calves are stiff and tight, it can change the entire mechanics of this very common movement and put undue stress through various parts of the body, including the knees and spine.

It's worth taking the time to test the mobility of each of these joints in turn, being careful as you do so. If you find any pain, stiffness or tightness as you do so, don't worry - after all, none of us are perfect - but you should certainly make a commitment to put in the work to improve the movement-specific mobility of this area of your body. Your body is one of your greatest assets and you need to make sure you look after it; after all, you only get one!

What Is Strength?

Throughout this book, one of the attributes we're going to talk about, possibly more than any other, is strength. By strength, I'm referring to the capability of a group of muscles within your body to produce force and therefore movement. Without strength, movement is impossible.

Strength is key, especially for over-fifties. Being strong protects you from injury as your joints will be far better supported against the effects of gravity. You'll be less likely to experience pain with arthritis. You'll be far less likely to fall, and less likely to suffer a life-changing injury as a result. You'll feel safer when you're out of the house and your confidence will grow as a result. You'll be able to do more around the home without worrying about paying for it the next day.

There really are no downsides to being strong and it is one of the greatest gifts I can give to my clients when I help them get strong enough to cope with the demands of their active lives.

So, how much strength do you really need to be healthy, fit and to remain active past the age of fifty? There are individual factors, including your daily routine, hobbies and goals, that determine the answer to this question. However, everyone needs a base level of strength to cope with the daily demands of life, unless you plan on becoming a couch potato until you pass away!

Being able to lift a suitcase over your head is a great indicator of upper body strength for over-fifties. If you can carry out this task, necessary as you board the plane bound for your next holiday of course, without undue stress or strain, it's likely that you've got good strength in your arms and shoulders.

Being able to go from standing to sitting in a low chair very slowly, without using your hands or letting yourself "drop" the last three inches into the chair, is a fantastic indicator of lower body strength. Although most of us get up and down from chairs every single day, it's incredible how much we use our upper body without realising in order to help us, sparing our legs… AND causing them to become weaker as a result! We are also inclined to drop quickly into chairs, relinquishing control to gravity, which causes us to quickly lose control of this movement even if we tried.

You should also have no problem walking on your tiptoes if asked to do so. This action proves lower body strength and demonstrates strong and capable feet and ankles.

These movements are some of the key indicators I use to test the strength of my clients. If they struggle to carry out these common, everyday actions aged fifty-five, how hard is life going to be at eighty?

But if you can't complete these actions without stress and strain on your body, it's not too late to do something about it. While muscle mass may continue to be lost with each advancing year, strength can be gained and maintained through practice and commitment. My aim is to show you how to do exactly that in this book.

What Is Endurance?

Endurance is your staying power. Having substantial endurance is a pre-requisite for being able to participate in daily life. If you have poor endurance, it's impossible to walk, run or cycle as far as you'd like. Endurance is determined by how efficient your lungs and heart are, as well as how much capacity for repetitive work your muscles house within them.

Why is endurance important?

Well, for a start, it determines how far you're able to walk with friends and family. It dictates how much of the housework you can get done in any given period. It also determines how likely you are to suffer an injury, to a certain extent. It can even be used to predict the cardiovascular health of an individual and the consequential likelihood of a heart attack.

While endurance usually refers to cardiovascular activity (the type of exercise that gets the heart pumping and the lungs working hard), we can also apply it to daily tasks, such as building a new piece of furniture or even cleaning your house.

A key point to consider about endurance is that it is very task-specific. For example, if you take a marathon runner, who is incredibly fit and has excellent running endurance, and put them on a bike, you may be surprised at how poorly they perform. The same is true for us and our daily tasks. We become very efficient at the things we do often - but not quite so good at new tasks that we don't know well, even if those tasks look simple at first glance.

How much endurance is enough to live a healthy life? The answer to this question is determined by your daily routine and the way you choose to live your life. Someone who runs three times per week will need more endurance than someone who just wants to maintain their garden. However, it is important to ensure that you maintain a baseline level of fitness that is sufficient for you to cope with the stresses and strains of daily life.

One way to improve your endurance is to simply add a little more activity onto the end of what you normally do, each time you do it. Endurance is built progressively and very slowly, just like building strength by working a specific muscle over and over again. If you want to be fitter so you can walk further or get more done each day, you need to first work out how much you can do within your current capacity. How much activity does it take until you feel like you have to stop, or until you feel like you're out of breath? This is your current endurance capacity.

If you want to improve your endurance capacity, the most sensible protocol goes something like this: next time you're out walking or doing jobs around the home, add five minutes on to the end of what you'd normally do before stopping. When you feel the call of a sit down on the sofa and a cup of tea, spur yourself on to do just five more minutes. If you're walking, take a slightly longer route than you normally would, but one that adds no more than five minutes onto your total walking time. Alternatively, you could try to walk roughly five percent quicker compared with the speed at which you usually walk.

By adding five extra minutes or five percent more effort to your current level of activity, you can slowly, incrementally build your staying power so that it's there to call on in the future, when you may absolutely need it. Having a solid level of endurance might be the difference between catching that flight and missing it altogether if you happen to be caught in awful traffic on the way to the airport. It might be the difference between getting across the road safely, or stumbling, at the end of a long walk. It might be the difference between a happy, tail-wagging pup and a sulking so-and-so after you tell the poor dog you can't take him out for a walk tonight because you're *just too tired.*

Building endurance takes time and a concerted effort, but once you start to reap the rewards, you'll feel such a difference. Imagine being able to climb that hill without getting out of breath; getting to the top of a long flight of stairs without feeling like your heart is going to burst out of your chest. Getting to the end of the day and feeling tired - but far from exhausted. These are the pay-offs for your hard work.

You'll also find benefits that aren't necessarily detectable by you, but will make a huge difference to your health. An improvement in heart health can lead to a dramatic decrease in the likelihood of suffering a fatal heart attack. It can prevent build-up of plaque in your arteries which could lead to problems like stroke. Improving your endurance is like taking out an insurance policy on your overall health. Being fitter is directly correlated with a reduced risk of not just cardiovascular problems, but of certain types of cancer[1] and even brain disorders like dementia[2].

So, the next time you're out for that weekend walk, try pushing yourself a little bit harder. Your heart, lungs and indeed the rest of your entire body will thank you for it!

Key Fundamental Movements (The Nine at Ninety!)

When you consider the things we have to do every day, there are a handful of common, yet highly challenging, movements we need to perform on a regular basis. After careful deliberation, I've compiled a list of the nine movements that I feel everyone should still be able to perform at age ninety to give you the best chance of a healthy body and incredible longevity!

If you have the ability to do every one of these activities without pain or restriction, it'll be unlikely that you'll be faced with anything in day-to-day life that you cannot handle. So, in no particular order, here are the nine key fundamental human movements - the *Nine at Ninety* - that, if maintained throughout your life, will make no physical challenge insurmountable!

1) The Chair Squat (with load)

This is an action we perform every single day, multiple times, yet most of us find incredibly imaginative ways to cheat. This causes us to miss out on the benefits of performing the action properly, and we lose the ability to perform it easily when required, as a result. What movement am I talking about? Getting in and out of a chair, of course!

Common cheating patterns usually appear in two ways:

1. Using our hands as leverage on well-placed chair arms.

2. Dropping into the chair on the way down.

So, as the first fundamental movement, my challenge to you is to be able to sit down and stand up from a low chair, one that puts your knees at a 90 degree angle when sitting, without the use of your hands. To make things harder but more effective, you're going to do so while holding something in front of your body. The reason you'll be holding something (preferably with a load of around 10% of your bodyweight) in front of your body is to add resistance - as well as to busy your hands and prevent you from reaching for those chair arms!

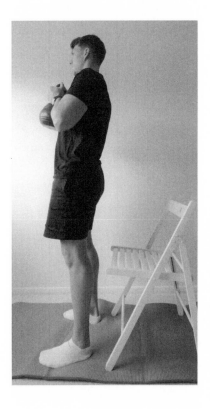
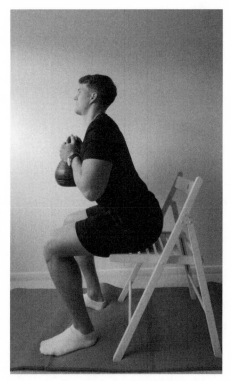

Why this movement is key: Being able to sit down and stand up with good control throughout this motion, without using your hands, shows excellent control of your thigh muscles - one of the key muscle groups for many tasks we perform every day. I use this movement as my number one quick screening tool when I have a client with a lower limb problem to check how well they're moving before we get to work.

2) The Suitcase Lift

Going on holiday is a wonderful time, and something we look forward to for many months prior to the trip. But holidaying can bring about a host of challenges that we don't often face at other times of the year. One of such challenges is lugging about a heavy suitcase, especially if you're going away for a period longer than one week (or you happen to have the packing habits of my girlfriend!)

We are forced to manoeuvre our suitcases in various ways around the airport and into transfer vehicles, which can be made easier by readily available assistance. However, one task that many of my clients hate relinquishing to others is the job of depositing the carry-on luggage into the over-head storage compartment on an aeroplane. Passing the task of lifting your wife's suitcase to the young buck in the seat behind, in front of a plane-full of people, can feel embarrassing.

By building enough strength to ensure you can complete this action, you're not only able to maintain your own independence in these matters but also help others less fortunate with their physical capabilities than you are. Suddenly, you'll transform into the one eagerly offering help to the cabin around you and not paying for it the next day.

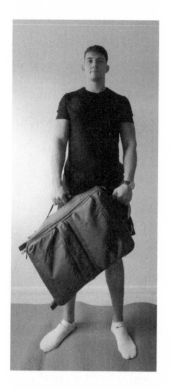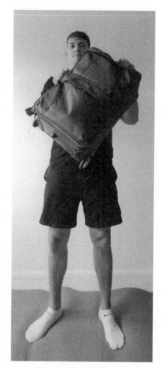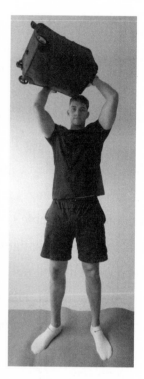

Why this movement is key: Being able to lift your luggage over your head and deposit it safely and securely, then retrieve it upon landing, is a feat that requires considerable upper body strength and stability. The shoulders, arms and "core" muscles are all highly active when we lift and shift above our heads, not to mention the need to satisfy the prerequisite of excellent shoulder mobility when it comes to reaching for your case. If you can lift a heavy case overhead in a tightly packed aeroplane and stow it away, ly, there probably aren't many overhead tasks that you'll find in daily life that will cause you a great deal of trouble.

3) The Stair Climb (with load)

For most people, stairs are a daily obstacle that we are forced to navigate. This is a good thing; stairs keep our legs strong and our joints mobile. I always fear for my clients when they downgrade from a house to a bungalow, as they'll lose the 10+ trips up the stairs each day and miss out on clocking up valuable minutes of strengthening exercise as a result.

However, being able to climb the stairs is only half the battle. It's important to be able to climb the stairs without the use of the handrail when one isn't available. It's also important to be able to transport a heavy load in each hand up and down the staircase when required. A great example of a load that we have to regularly transfer up and down stairs are bags of heavy shopping. We might buy a new lamp or want to decorate the bedroom, or we might even have an upstairs kitchen. Either way, getting load up stairs independently is an important job we regularly have to do.

Why this movement is key: If you think about the way we climb stairs, we must put all of our weight on one leg when we transfer from one step to another. This requires balance and single-leg stability, which is vital for many of our other daily tasks. We also need to use our thigh muscles to their maximum capability to control our descent down a flight of stairs, more so than when we walk on the flat. Climbing the stairs with a bag of shopping in each hand is a great acid test for your leg strength and overall stability. If you can do this task, it should bring you confidence across the board.

4) The Floor Get-Up

One of the things I am most proud of when it comes to the treatment I offer in my clinic is that I regularly help my clients to avoid the terrifying prospect of a fall. Falling can be catastrophic for anyone, but especially for people over the age of seventy. Falls cost the NHS over £1billion per year, purely because of the extent of the physical damage that can occur from the impact. Coupled with the fact that fallers are more likely to have fragile bones than the general population, the perils of suffering a fall are great and should be prevented at all costs where possible.

However, some of us are going to fall at some stage in our lives. Luckily, for many people falls don't damage anything more than their confidence, but having fallen there is another problem you must face immediately after. That problem is how to get up from the floor, especially when no one else is around.

The NHS guidelines, taught to us in my hospital placement days, recommended the use of a chair to pull on to go from lying to kneeling, then the use of that same chair to push up onto to go from kneeling to standing. However, what happens when there are no chairs or other suitable pieces of furniture within reach? I've met more than one older person who fell in their home, and despite not being injured, had to wait for paramedics to arrive before they could get back onto their feet. This was a particularly distressing event for each of these people, and I wouldn't wish it on anyone.

That is why I believe being able to get up from the floor, without the use of a chair or any other piece of furniture to help, is one essential fundamental movement making up my *Nine at Ninety*. It is also the movement that may be considered the hardest of the nine movements, involving literally the entire body and a series of complex, coordinated actions.

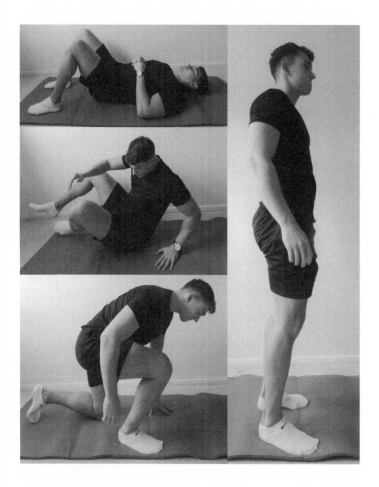

Why this movement is key: We've discussed why being able to get up from the floor is so critical, but what does it take to actually be able to get up and down from the floor? For a start, you need impressive "core" strength: the capability of your midriff to stabilise your body as you go from lying to sitting. You'll then need to be stable enough to swing a leg round and push up on it to go from sitting to kneeling. Once in a kneeling position, it takes a fair amount of leg strength to push up to standing without toppling over.

All in all, this is the ultimate movement - once you can achieve the Floor Get-Up, you'll have impressive confidence and should find the other fundamental movements on this list a piece of cake in comparison. A quick word about practicing this movement: if you choose to do so, be sure to start on a soft carpeted floor with someone supervising and plenty of furniture within reach to use to help you stand up if you get stuck.

5) The Hole Dig

Is there any task in the garden more physical than digging a great big hole? Digging holes can be an incredibly satisfying activity and one that I always used to love participating in on the rare occasion that I would help my Mum in the garden.

Digging a hole isn't just a necessary part of transforming a garden, though; it's also a great marker of strength and endurance. Digging with a heavy spade is an activity that involves a range of muscle groups, meaning the benefits of this activity are widespread too. You'll probably notice yourself getting breathless as you dig the hole. This shows how the cardiovascular system is also being called upon to join in and is strengthened as a result.

Why this movement is key: When digging a hole, you'll need both upper and lower body strength. Not only will each thrust of the spade require a maximal effort from your muscles, but the effort will require your heart and lungs to be working well in combination too. Because of this, being able to dig a hole represents the ability to perform a truly practical, physical activity that transfers across many other DIY or garden tasks.

6) The Five-Mile Walk

So far, we've discussed movements that require a lot of explosive strength and impressive mobility. But what is the activity we do the most each day, that also happens to be the number one hobby of thousands of over-fifties? The answer to that question is: walking.

Being able to walk without discomfort is an absolute necessity for a happy, healthy life. Experts have long believed that getting 10,000 steps in each day (the truth about that later in the book) is an effective way of mitigating the risk of many health problems; but how many of us have the capacity to do that number of steps all in one go?

The ability to walk five miles is a great indicator of excellent general mobility and endurance. Being able to walk this far opens up a whole new list of possibilities for social activities, as well as giving you licence to explore some of the beautiful natural treats the countryside has to offer.

Why this movement is key: You can think of walking over a medium-to-long distance as a good audit of your general mobility. Over this type of distance, little niggles and problems with your walking technique are likely to show; highlighting areas of your body that need extra work. What's more, having the ability to walk five miles gives you confidence in certain situations that, luckily, we don't have to contend with very often but are always a possibility - such as being stranded somewhere far flung after your car has broken down, with no signal to call the *AA*.

7) The Gardening Crouch

This movement isn't limited solely to the garden, although it is possibly the time when you need it most. The gardening crouch describes the process of squatting down and sitting back on your haunches in order to reach something low to the ground. You would also need this movement in situations such as reaching for something in a low cupboard in your kitchen. Imagine you have to pull a weed up from the ground but you don't want to get your knees muddy. You're going to need to crouch down while remaining supported on two feet. This is the gardening crouch.

The gardening crouch is primarily a marker of good mobility. It requires excellent mobility of your ankles, knees and hips to be able to hold it comfortably. The common substitute people make for this movement when they lack proper mobility in their lower limbs is to "fold" at the waist and use the movement of their lower back to reach for the floor. While not necessarily harmful to do once or twice, constant repetitive use of this action can lead to back pain and likely isn't good for long-term back health.

By instead using the gardening crouch, your weight is going through your ankles, knees and hips, which are much better designed to tolerate the load of your body. The easiest way to tell whether or not you are capable of the gardening crouch is to think back to the last time you were transferring a small plant from a pot to the garden, or when you needed something out of a low cupboard - what did you do to get down there? Did you bend at the waist while keeping your legs straight? Did you sit on the floor? Did you go down onto your knees?

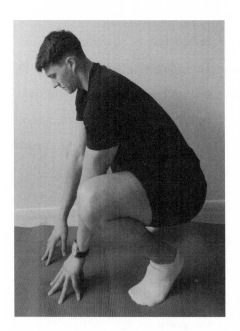 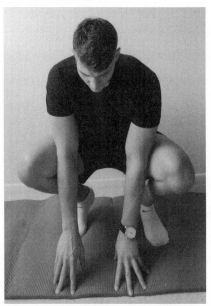

If you did any of those things instead of the gardening crouch, you may lack mobility in one or two of the key joints in your legs. Don't worry - we'll talk later in this book about how to improve the movement in those joints if they are indeed limited.

Why this movement is key: This movement is part of the Nine at Ninety because it demonstrates excellent hip, knee and ankle health. One cannot put their entire bodyweight through their fully-bent knees if the knees are deteriorated, stiff or unhealthy. While some strength is involved, this movement really tests the mobility of the lower limb, more so than the other movements on this list.

8) The Box Lift

Being able to pick up a heavy object from very low down on the floor is a vital ability to retain in advancing years. First, let's picture the movement; imagine a heavy box in your front room that needs moving into the kitchen. To pick it up you must bend down, at the waist and the knees, gripping the box around the lower edges and then extending your back and knees so as to lift it up and carry it away.

To do so, you'll need sufficient grip strength to get started. Being able to use your fingers and hands effectively is incredibly important at any stage of your life. There are chapters on how to maintain the use of your hands later in this book.

You'll also need to use proper lifting technique to perform this exercise well. There is in fact a "right" way to lift, a way that will use the full potential of your leg and back muscles while also mitigating the risk of injury. You'll need to also use the strength in your back and legs to perform this movement properly, protecting your back while safely lifting the box into your arms.

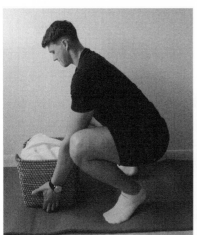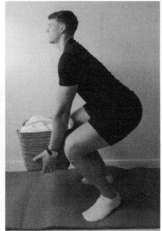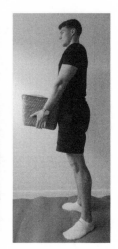

Why this movement is key: We have to lift things from the floor quite often. Fortunately for us, most things that we lift are light and can be moved relatively safely, regardless of technique. However, when we come across a heavy load firmly planted on the floor that needs shifting, it's important we have the ability to do this without putting ourselves at risk of injury. For this movement, ankle and hip mobility are vital, as well as strength and coordination of the lower limb muscles. Without all of these prerequisites, we'll be putting ourselves at unnecessary risk.

9) The Wood Chop

The final movement in the *Nine at Ninety* is one that not many of us have to do with any regularity, but one that highlights strength, stability and mobility almost better than any other.

This movement is the wood chop. Think of a lumberjack chopping wood on a block, swinging an axe overhead and bringing it down with incredible accuracy onto a semi-split log. While I'm not suggesting that you go to a hardware store and purchase the largest axe you can find, some of you reading this chapter may still chop wood in this way. Even if you don't, I think it is important to consider just how many different areas of the body need to work in tandem to produce such a primal movement. Once you have a mental picture of the demands this task involves, you can decide whether it is something that is within your capabilities or not.

Chopping wood requires you to generate the force to swing the axe first with your lower limbs, then transfer the force up through your trunk into your arms, before contracting your shoulders and trunk to bring the axe down. In this way, almost every muscle group in the body is used in a chain reaction.

Why this movement is key: As previously mentioned, this task isn't something most of us have to do very often, but it is a fantastic "movement audit" for the whole body. You'll need strength in both upper and lower limbs, as well as excellent mobility in the spine, hips and shoulders to perform this movement effectively. If you can safely chop wood at ninety and beyond, you'll be doing incredibly well!

What To Do With The *Nine at Ninety*

If you've considered the movements I describe above and think that most of these are within your capabilities at this current time, that is fantastic and should be applauded. Your task is simply to *maintain* your ability to perform these movements as each year passes, watching out for early signs of stiffness or weakness that may prohibit your movement.

Key "sticky" areas to watch for are loss of movement in your shoulder joints, tightness in your calves and stiffness in the hips and knees. Keep an eye on these areas and seek guidance if you feel stiffness or tightness setting in any time soon.

If you can't complete the tasks in the *Nine at Ninety*, don't worry; it's likely that you're just out of practice. When we don't use these parts of our body regularly, we lose the ability to call on them when we need them. But, in many cases, this process is reversible! With some targeted work or treatment from a skilled professional, there are many goals that are closer to being within reach than you think.

First, you need to work out if the reason that you can't perform these movements is because of lack of practice, or because of an injury preventing you from doing so. My recommendations would be to first get the injury problem solved before trying to push on with these tasks. Seek out some professional advice about your individual circumstances.

Once your injury has improved, look for the strength and mobility advice within this book, which will demonstrate the ways that you can improve your movement, taking you ever closer to being able to safely perform the *Nine at Ninety*.

One of the key things to remember is that improving strength and mobility takes a long time! You're likely to be several months, at a minimum, away from your goals. However, just a short period of time dedicated to solving these problems each day will go a long way to improving your capability in these actions and many more that you carry out each day.

Now, in the following pages of this book, we're going to talk about specific areas of the body, one by one. My hope is that in each chapter, you'll learn something useful that you can apply to your own life or routine in order to improve your health, fitness and longevity. Let's get started with the head, neck and shoulders.

CHAPTER TWO

Head, Neck & Shoulders

Introduction

In this chapter, I'm going to share my stories, expert information and best guidance for problems involving the head, the neck and the shoulders. In my clinic, I regularly help people not just with painful necks and shoulders, but also headaches as well. The problems are often linked; for example, it's common to find that when a client's neck pain is treated, their headaches disappear too.

In this chapter, you'll find out the best sleeping positions, best time to get a massage, how to ease a stiff neck, the truth about your posture, and much more.

The problems we talk about in this chapter are incredibly common; so if you're suffering with one of these issues, don't panic! You're certainly not alone.

Get a cup of tea or coffee, get comfortable, and let's start by talking about what we can do to stop headaches in their tracks.

Could It Be Your NECK Giving You Headaches?

Headaches are an incredibly common problem. In fact, 3 out of every 4 adults in the UK will suffer to some degree from recurrent headaches.

For some, this pain can be daily and extremely debilitating.

For those who do suffer with frequent headaches, my first thought would be to try and help them identify the underlying cause of their headache. We would start by asking them to try to explain the characteristics of their headache.

Is it like a tight band around the head? Is it just at the back of the head, or does it go all over? Does it feel like a pulsing pain is present behind the eyes?

All of these questions can help to pinpoint the root cause of a headache (which is paramount for treating it).

Now, not many people know this, but many headaches in adults are caused by problems in the neck. We call these '*cervicogenic headaches*'.

Have you ever suffered from a stiff neck with pain radiating up into the back of your head? If you have, you'll know just how unpleasant a headache like this can be. Some of my clients tell me a headache like this is much worse than the neck pain they started with!

The interesting thing is that it is also possible to suffer from cervicogenic headaches without feeling any neck pain whatsoever. This can make it very hard to tell whether the neck is responsible or if the culprit is something else entirely.

Here are a few clues which can help you identify a neck-related headache:

- You might feel the headache at the back of the head, on one or both sides, or it could be round the sides of the head too. Less common is pain behind the eyes or across the forehead.
- Your headache might get worse when you turn your head, like when you drive or turn to speak to someone.
- The headache will usually be more like a dull ache than a sharp pain.
- You might also have some neck pain too, although this isn't always the case.

The cause behind these neck-related headaches is usually the fact that either the muscles are very tight in the neck, or the joints aren't moving quite as well as they should be for one of a few reasons.

Be sure to get any new, persistent headache assessed by your doctor first, but here are some top tips to help with this problem at home:

- **Keep your neck mobile!** The stiffer it gets, the worse the headache. Moving your neck might initially make the pain a little worse, but it should get better in the long run with some gentle movement within a comfortable range.

- **Use heat treatment on your neck.** Applying a warm compress to the back of your neck for 15-minutes at a time (be sure to protect the skin) can help to ease tight muscles and loosen stiff joints. Even if the pain is only in the head, this will often still help!

• **Try the exercise in the next section of this book** (*"Relieve Neck Pain & Stiffness with One Exercise"*) for pain relief and to restore range of motion in your neck, providing it's safe for you to do so.

• **Your sleeping position is important.** If lying on your side, your neck and head should be in line with your shoulders, as if you were upright. Try to experiment with an extra pillow, or take one away if you currently use more than one, to see if that improves matters. Sometimes, getting a new pillow might be a good idea. If you sleep on your back, use a supportive pillow and a rolled towel at the back of the neck, as shown in the picture below.

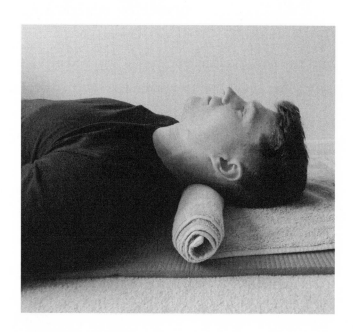

- **Try to watch your posture.** By gently pulling your shoulder blades back and down when you sit (rather than rounding your shoulders) you can often relieve some of the stress in tired neck muscles and improve your headaches as a result. Try to imagine your lower back, mid-back, shoulders and head stacked atop one another and balancing there when you're sat.

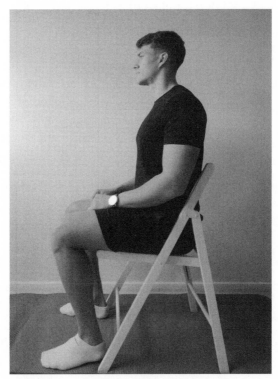

Although no posture is "perfect", good sitting posture can be maintained by imagining everything "stacked" on top of each other when sitting.

Relieve Neck Pain & Stiffness with ONE Exercise!

By far, one of the most common questions I get asked by the people who come to see me in my clinic is the following: *"How do I get rid of this damn stiff neck?!"*

Most of the time, that person has either slept in a strange position and woken up stiff, or they just felt a tweak in their neck one day that led to it 'stiffening up' over a number of days.

Either way, they aren't happy! And I don't blame them. Neck pain is, well, a pain in the neck!

Luckily, we're usually able to give these people a great solution to their neck pain. It works especially well for people over fifty, as the root cause of their neck pain is often something we call a 'joint dysfunction'. That's a fancy term for a situation where the joints in the neck aren't quite moving as they should be.

You see, you've got seven bones in your neck and the way they work is quite intricate. They all move in an organised fashion, articulating with one another, powered by the tiny muscles that surround them.

If for some reason that movement becomes imbalanced, the body senses a problem and goes on red alert.

The way your body then acts to 'protect' you from harm is to tighten up and the brain causes you to feel pain. Pain is simply a signal from the body that says *"Don't move, it's not safe!"* On the surface level, this might seem like a stupid response to simply sleeping in a strange position one night, but it's actually very clever. Your brain isn't able to differentiate between true damage and perceived damage. It can't be sure you haven't suffered a serious injury. So, in order to prevent you from suffering further injury, it causes you so much pain and stiffness that you aren't able to move that body part any more until it heals.

So, even though you haven't damaged anything, your neck is still stiff and sore! How are we supposed to fix it?

The answer is, we have to show the body that it's safe to move again. And the exercise below will help you do exactly that.

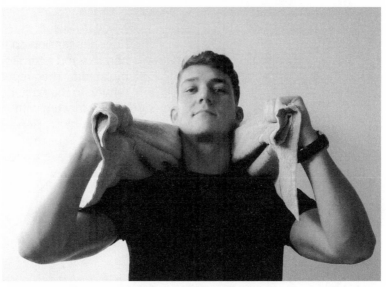

Start by rolling a hand towel lengthways into a band. Place the band around the back of your neck, near where the head meets the neck. Pull firmly forward so as to add tension to the towel.

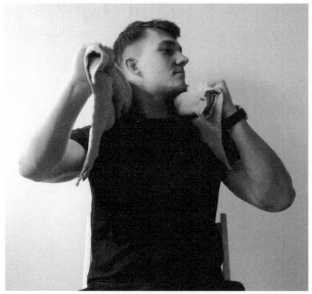

Keeping tension on the towel throughout, as you turn your head to the left, pull forwards with your right hand. You might find that you are able to turn your head further than you normally can.

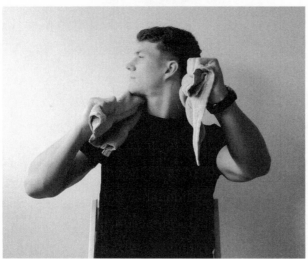

Keep the tension on the band as you return to the centre. Then repeat turning to the right, but pulling forward with your left hand. Repeat 10 times in each direction, several times each day.

A Natural Approach to Treating Migraines

I remember throughout my childhood, there would sometimes be whole days, even weeks, where my mother couldn't get out of bed.

She could barely even open her eyes or speak during these episodes. I didn't fully understand it at the time; why was she behaving so strangely?

It wasn't until I was old enough to understand that she told me that these terrible times were caused by migraines.

Anyone who's suffered with a migraine will be able to tell you how debilitating they can be. Which is why it can be nothing short of infuriating when someone dares to compare them to a simple headache!

There are several medications available that are designed to treat migraines and, for most people, they are sufficient to reduce the frequency or intensity of the suffering. But for many, these medications don't solve the underlying cause.

What is often missed is an imbalance in the body somewhere, causing these chronic migraines. Your migraines could actually be caused by a deficiency in certain vitamins and minerals, or an intolerance to a common food in your diet.

My initial advice to anyone coming to me with migraines is to first get the levels of vitamins and minerals in their blood tested. You can get relatively inexpensive vitamin and mineral blood tests online, or ask your doctor for one.

Magneisum, vitamin-B and co-enzyme Q10 supplements have been shown to help migraines in some promising clinical trials[1]. This book is all about finding natural ways to treat even the most stubborn issues; if you're fed up with taking medication for your migraines this may be something you want to read more about and discuss with your doctor to see if it is suitable for you to try.

Something you should bear in mind is that migraines have been linked consistently with hormonal fluctuations. We all know about 'the change' that women of a certain age go through, so speaking to your doctor about balancing your hormones if they are running amok can often go a long way to fixing the issue at its root cause.

Failing that, the thing that worked for my mother was an elimination diet. She slowly cut out various suspect foods from her diet until she found two clear triggers for her awful migraines: cocoa and coffee.

Unfortunately, her body didn't care that these were her favourite treats. However, she wouldn't hesitate to say that cutting these foods from her diet was worth the return to normality, without persistent, 72-hour-long migraines.

Why You Need More Than Massage to Fix Your Neck Pain

One thing that took me a long time to understand when it comes to pain is the fact that the painful area isn't always the source of the problem. This is never truer than with neck pain.

When I first started my career as a physiotherapist, when people would come to see me about their neck pain they would point to their neck and say *"this is where it hurts"*. Diligently, I would provide treatment and exercises, all targeted at the painful area. For some, I'd get good results.

However, for many, they would only get temporary relief. They'd tell me how the exercises work… *for about five minutes*. Then it's back to square one.

I couldn't understand how I wasn't making progress with these people in my first year of practice. It wasn't until another year or so that I realised I wasn't *treating* the problem at all. I was simply *masking* the surface-level problem. My methods back then were on par with pain killers; concealing the symptoms without resolving the underlying cause.

A paradigm-shifting moment came for me when I started to address not just the symptoms but the driving force behind the neck complaint.

The truth is, for many people who suffer from neck pain when sitting, driving or working, there will be a group of muscles that are working far too hard. This tends to be the painful region. Why are these muscles working too hard? The reason is because there is usually another group of muscles somewhere in the vicinity *not working hard enough*. These lazy muscles aren't doing their job properly, so the stronger muscles in the neck decide to take over. They think *"if those lazy muscles aren't doing their job, I guess I'm going to have to pick up the slack!"*

And that's where the problem starts. These stronger, overworked muscles are now doing two jobs instead of the one job they were designed to do. So it's no wonder they start to complain after a while. And when a muscle complains, it gives you pain.

So, let's bring it back to the treatment room. If I were to massage your tight, tired muscles - the ones that are doing all the work - it might make them feel good for a while. But as soon as you start to move again, they still have to pick up the slack from the other muscles that have effectively 'switched off'.

This means that we need to take a different approach to treating neck pain. We can't just rub the painful area and expect the pain not to come back. How easy life would be if that were true!

What we need to do instead is to encourage the lazy muscles in our neck and upper body to start working a bit harder, to start doing their job again, rather than passing the buck to the all-too-eager muscles that end up over-worked and in pain.

The next few sections of this book are dedicated to giving you a few strategies for doing just that. Sure, the techniques on the following pages are useful *alongside* massage. But never rely on massage alone to get that neck better!

Instead, let's have a look at some better strategies…

The Truth About Posture

When a physiotherapist starts to talk about neck pain, everyone expects that the next line to come out of their mouth will be something along the lines of: *"...And you need to watch your posture!"*

It's become very expected from a physiotherapy session and many of my clients glumly admit to me that they have "poor posture", even before I've assessed them.

But what exactly *is* poor posture?

Is poor posture just slouching? Or is there more to it than that?

My definition of "poor posture" is simply a position that is suboptimal for the performance of a given task, whether that be sitting, standing or walking. This means that poor posture, in fact, must always be assessed in context of the task at hand.

To make matters more complicated, as humans we are all built differently to one another. Some of us have long legs and a short body, while others have long spines or even a leg length difference. This means that *your* so-called "perfect posture" is going to be completely different to that of your neighbour for any given task.

However, there are some general rules to follow that apply to all; for example, it makes sense to sit and stand in a way that puts the least stress on our joints and muscles.

One of the ways we can do this is through ensuring that when we sit or stand, we try to maintain a position where the structures in our neck and shoulders are "stacked" on top of one another. This is the best way to avoid excess mechanical stress or tension on these parts of our body.

There are two great "cues" you can use that I've found to help you do this. One helps when you stand and walk, while the other helps while sitting.

Now that almost all of us use computers, laptops, tablets and phones every day, a great proportion of our day is spent looking at the gadget in our hand or on our laps, sitting about 12 inches away from our face. The use of these gadgets encourages us to poke our chins forward as we strain to see small print, and round our shoulders as we use our hands to type. These subtle postural changes take our neck and shoulders out of "alignment" and put undue stress on weaker muscles. It's no wonder that people who work office jobs, or spend a lot of time on social media, are far more likely to suffer neck pain than their more active counterparts.

When we get up after a prolonged laptop session, the muscles that became shortened during our time spent sitting don't automatically return to their normal length. This means that we tend to remain in this new poor posture even after our computer sessions, staying in a suboptimal posture when we get up to walk around again unless we consciously do something about it.

The first step to correcting this issue is simply to be aware that it's happening.

Once you're aware of it, you can ask yourself *"are my shoulders tipped forward and rounded? Is my chin poking forward?"*

If the answer to any of these questions is a "yes", then you can make very subtle changes to take the pressure off these key areas again.

One way to do this is to imagine that your sternum (the hard bone that sits in the middle of your chest) is a small but very full glass of water.

When you walk around with your shoulders rounded, your sternum tends to be tilted forward. If you imagine your sternum being a full glass of water, I want you to imagine the water within it spilling out and trickling down your front.

Now, to stop the spillage: slightly pull your shoulders back and push your chest out a little. Notice how your sternum tilts back - it should be perfectly upright now, and the water stays in the glass. Use this visualisation whenever you get up after being sat on a laptop or phone for any length of time.

To improve your posture while walking, there is another great visualisation I commonly teach my clients. If you imagine a piece of string attached to the top of your head, picture what would happen if a magical force from above pulled on the string to make you as tall as possible. You'd feel yourself grow an inch, your chest would come out and your shoulders would move backwards slightly too. This would happen to be an excellent posture to maintain while walking to take pressure off the neck and mid-back. These slight tweaks can offer an effective solution to pain in these areas.

Re-Engage Those Lazy Muscles

In the previous chapter, we spoke about how to become more aware of what "good posture" is and how to avoid spending too much time in suboptimal postures. That alone will go some way to taking strain and tension away from your neck and shoulders.

However, we still need to work on re-engaging the muscles around your neck and shoulders that have effectively 'switched off'. These lazy muscles have shrugged their workload onto their bigger, stronger cousins so that they can take to the back seat and enjoy a free ride.

What we're going to do in this chapter is learn exactly how to kick-start these commonly lazy muscles and have them pick up the slack again!

The muscles we are going to work on strengthening sit between your shoulder blades. They are responsible for keeping your shoulders in good alignment as you perform delicate tasks using your arms (such as using a mouse or keyboard).

You'll need a light resistance band for the exercise on the following page. You can get these very cheaply online or from your local sports store. You won't need much resistance to start off with, so get the thinnest one you can find to practice with first.

Once you've got your resistance band, you're going to do the following:

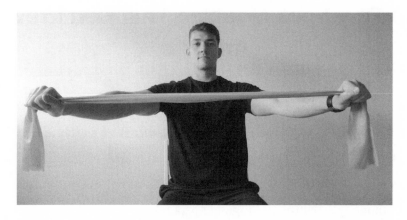

Hold it in both hands with your palms facing down, with some slack in the band between your hands. Raise your arms up straight in front of you so that they come up to chest level. Don't let your shoulders 'shrug' up towards your ears; keep them relaxed and low.

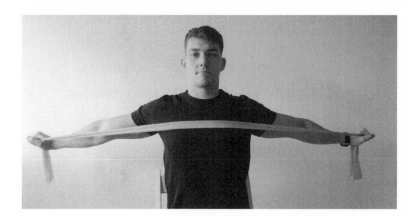

Keeping your shoulders relaxed and low, pull the band apart as far as you possibly can, by engaging the muscles between your shoulder blades. Once you've pulled the band right across your chest, make every effort to squeeze your shoulder blades together even more, as if you're trying to pinch a pencil between them. Hold this position for 3-5 seconds. Slowly let the band return to the start position in front of your chest. *Repeat this exercise until you get a slight working ache between your shoulder blades, or until you can't stop your shoulders from shrugging up towards your ears; whichever comes first.*

The Tiny Neck Muscles That Can Prevent Arthritis

The human neck is an incredible example of nature's architecture at its finest. One of the most complex areas of the human body, the neck houses intricate bony structures, branches and bundles of nerves and muscles that work both independently and together as a unit.

As we spoke about earlier in this book, our necks tend to feel better if we sit and stand in a way that puts us in a position where all the structures within the neck are properly 'stacked up' on top of each other.

Think of it like a game of *Jenga* - if you stack the blocks correctly, the tower is stable. However, if you stack them in a rush, with some of the little wooden blocks skew-whiff, your tower is no longer as stable and is instead prone to stress and strain. Our necks are no different.

We can't change the bones in our neck. They are largely innate and we inherited them when we were born. However, what we can change is the pulling force on these bones by asking certain muscles to do the correct amount of work. This is the way to limit stress and strain on the tiny joints in our necks, regardless of the anatomy that nature endowed us with.

One of the reasons we definitely want to limit undue stress and strain on our intricate neck joints is that it helps to prevent arthritis. "Arthritis" is a term used to describe the wearing down of the cartilage within our joints, and I'll refer to it many times throughout the course of this book.

Even if you've been told that you already have some arthritis in your neck, this need not be cause for concern necessarily. The exercises we use to prevent the problem are usually the exact same ones we might use to treat it, so this chapter can still help.

There exists a group of tiny muscles that live within your neck, under your chin. They are given the daunting task of supporting your head when you sit, walk and move.

In order to support the weight of the head (which is enormous in comparison to the size of these tiny muscles), it is vital that these muscles are able to do their job well, no matter how small they might be.

So, how do we know if these tiny muscles are working as they were designed?

If you find that the back of your neck aches after you've been driving any distance, or you've noticed that your chin pokes forward when you sit or walk, it's likely that these tiny neck muscles aren't doing their job very well at all. You might also notice a '*compressing*' feeling at the back of your neck, as if something is being trapped or crushed there. That feeling is the weight of your head putting strain on the joints in your neck, simply because your neck muscles aren't working as hard as they should.

If left untreated, this continuous pressure can cause problems later down the line.

But don't worry - we can fix it!

The exercise that follows is a fantastic way to resolve this 'crushing' sensation at the back of your neck, helping with neck pain, headaches and stiffness too. It's a very subtle exercise that doesn't require much effort;

just plenty of regularity and persistence. Lots of my patients find that they can quite happily get on with this exercise in front of the TV or in the car.

Here's how you can find the muscles we want to activate: from a sitting position, keep your eyes level and pull your chin in, as if to make a double chin. The muscles you can feel working are the ones we are going to target.

I usually recommend that you try to dedicate at least 10 minutes a day, split evenly into smaller chunks of time, to practicing this exercise if you're suffering from neck pain, or you'd like to take out an insurance policy against neck arthritis!

Here are the 3 simple steps:
• Start sitting upright somewhere comfortable with your eyes looking straight ahead (picture A, next page)
• Gently pull your chin in as if you're trying to make a very subtle double chin (picture B). Keep your eyes gazing straight ahead and don't let your nose move towards the floor as you do this.
• Hold this position for 5 seconds, then relax to your normal position. Repeat this for several minutes whenever sitting still for any length of time.

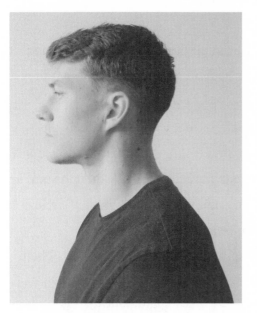

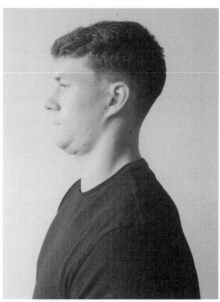

Picture A   Picture B

Counter the Effects of Sitting

It isn't just our necks that get stiff from all the sitting we do each and every day. There are other parts of our body that suffer, even though they tend not to complain quite so much.

One area that tends to be problematic for many of my clients is the mid-back, or thoracic spine. The surprising truth is that many people don't know that area of their body has become incredibly stiff. Although some get mid-back pain quite regularly, many don't - even though they've lost almost *all* of the movement in this important area of the trunk.

The mid-back is the region of the spine that allows you to twist. There isn't very much rotation available at your lower back, so even though you may feel like you're rotating at the lower back when you turn your torso, 90% of that movement is coming from the middle section of your spine.

It's also vital that we maintain another movement of the mid-back, called extension (otherwise known as leaning back). Being able to extend allows us to walk and stand without putting too much pressure on other areas of the body.

So, how can your mid-back become so stiff all of a sudden?

The real truth is: the process is not very sudden at all! The mid-back becomes stiff and restricted over a period of many years and there's one position that tends to be responsible for this. If you guessed that the position responsible for this stiffness is sitting, you're absolutely correct.

Being in a seated position increases the curvature in your spine, placing you in a flexed forward position. Being flexed forward is the opposite of extension or leaning back, so if we don't make an effort to do that action in order to counteract the many hours of sitting we do each day, we lose the ability to perform extension at all.

The old saying is absolutely true: **If you don't use it, you lose it!**

When we lose the ability to move freely, other areas need to pick up the slack. Quite often, it tends to be the neck that draws the short straw. This is why a lot of neck pain can actually be attributed to a stiff mid-back, rather than a problem with the neck itself.

Luckily, all is not lost, even if you've spent half your life working an office job. Yes, you'll be stiff, but you can also work to regain some of that lost movement.

The 2-minute routine below will help many with mid-back pain, as well as those who suffer from neck pain and even those who feel stiff in the neck or trunk when they sit or drive. I would recommend you do this routine before you sit or drive for any distance, or just whenever you feel a bit stiff and want a way to loosen up quickly.

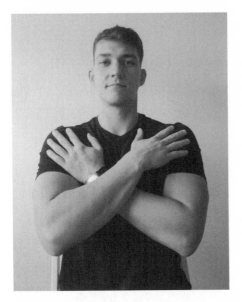

Start sitting in a chair with arms crossed over your chest. Turn first to the left (picture A), then to the right (picture B), slowly and carefully. Rotate right and left 10 times in a row x 3 per day.

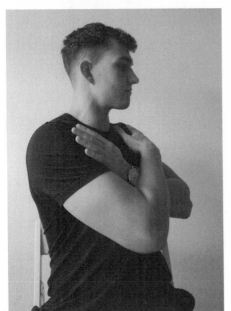

Picture A

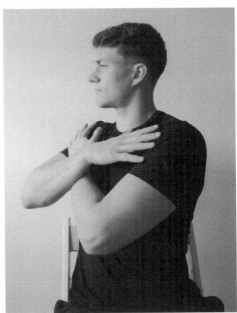

Picture B

Get Relief from a Frozen Shoulder

The dreaded frozen shoulder: intense pain, sleep disturbance and an inability to use one arm for absolutely no apparent reason, followed by months of debilitating stiffness. It's no wonder my patients groan when they get this diagnosis.

If you've been diagnosed with a frozen shoulder, or suspect you might have one, it's important to understand this condition a little better first.

Frozen shoulder is a problem that the medical world doesn't yet fully understand. We haven't identified an absolute trigger for what causes it yet[2], but we know there are some risk factors that make it more likely (such as being female, diabetic or having thyroid problems[3]).

A frozen shoulder starts with intense pain in the shoulder or upper arm. Over a number of weeks to months, that pain will reduce, and profound stiffness will take its place. And as quickly and mysteriously as it started, it will eventually disappear on its own as well.

If you're suffering at the moment from a frozen shoulder, it's important to know that you're not alone: around 3% of the population will go through this at some point in their lifetime[2].

Now, if your frozen shoulder is keeping you awake all night and getting in the way of your daily routine, it might be worth speaking to your doctor about pain relief, then getting some advice about whether the exercise below is suitable for you or not.

The exercise in this section is a very effective pain-reliever. It produces an effect called 'traction' on the shoulder joint, which basically means you're gently and safely pulling the shoulder joint apart and creating a nice 'gap' in the joint. This helps by allowing more lubricating *synovial fluid* into the joint - which reduces some of the constricting pressure in the shoulder and should give you much needed relief.

For this exercise, all you'll need is a small weight or dumbbell to hold, or, alternatively, you could use a rucksack or sturdy bag and fill it with some books.

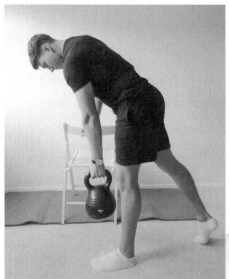

Start off holding a weight or a rucksack filled with some heavy books. Take support with your hand on a chair or worktop. Lean forward so that your affected shoulder is hanging down as shown.

Slowly start to swing the weight like a pendulum, forward and back. As you do this, try to let gravity do the work and let your shoulder relax as much as you can. Continue for 30-seconds x 2-3 per day.

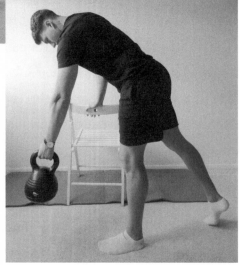

Defrost Your Frozen Shoulder

If you're suffering from a true frozen shoulder, the initial, excruciating pain should pass within a few months. However, what you will be left with is a shoulder that *really* doesn't want to move.

This is what gives frozen shoulder its name. I've had clients whose shoulders are literally pinned to their sides, hardly able to move the arm because it has seized up so severely. Anyone who has suffered from this condition will tell you that it isn't pain that's stopping them from moving their arm; it just physically *won't* go.

The reason for the arm being so stuck is that this condition causes the shoulder joint to effectively 'seize up' as the shoulder capsule becomes tight and constricted. The shoulder capsule is a fibrous wrapping encasing your entire shoulder joint. It keeps everything in place and stops the joint from being unstable in normal circumstances. However, in frozen shoulder, the capsule seizes up and becomes far tighter than it is designed to be. This significantly impedes mobility.

Although the research isn't conclusive as to whether lots of treatment can help to improve the mobility of a frozen shoulder[4], I always think having a great home exercise programme to improve mobility of the arm is a good idea. In my experience, the people who truly apply themselves to an exercise programme, or indeed get effective hands-on treatment, tend to have far better results than those who just sit and wait for this problem to go away on its own.

The exercise programme that follows will show you a few movements that you can do regularly to regain the movement and function of your arm. If you can dedicate ten minutes each day to practicing these movements, that should be sufficient for you to notice some improvement in how far you can put your arms over your head, how much you can lift, and how easy it is to reach that damn bra strap!

Be sure to check with your healthcare provider before starting any new exercise programme like this one, to make sure it is appropriate for you and your individual circumstances.

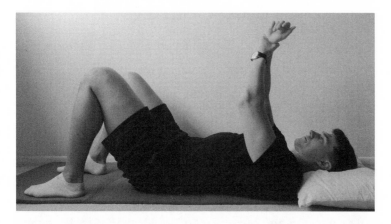

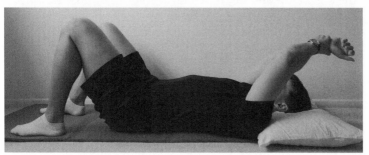

Grasp the wrist of your painful arm with your good hand. Using your good hand to help, take the painful arm over your head until you reach the feeling of resistance. Gently move into and out of this resistance using your good arm to help. Continue with this movement for 30-seconds x 4-5 per day for best results.

The Most Important Shoulder Muscles You Never Knew You Had

When we think about strong shoulder muscles, the first picture that springs to mind might be that of an enormous, towering body builder with boulders for shoulders. But the muscles that you can see on any behemoth body builder aren't the ones that you and I should be most concerned with.

There is a far more discrete set of muscles that are the origin of our impressive ability to throw, lift and climb, whilst also unfortunately being the source of a lot of suffering for many people. These small yet vital muscles are collectively called the '*rotator cuff*'.

The rotator cuff is comprised of four smaller muscles that sit around your shoulder blade and attaching onto the bone of your upper arm (called the humerus). These muscles have a very important job. They keep your shoulder in its socket, as well as stabilising your arm whenever you lift it away from your side.

The rotator cuff is so called because these four muscles converge to form one large tendon that resembles a 'cuff', attaching the muscles to the humerus. When it is in good working order, your rotator cuff is a phenomenal evolutionary feature of humankind. It allowed us to hunt, once upon a time, and being able to accurately throw projectiles gave humans the edge, even over some of the most formidable predators that cohabited the prehistoric world with us.

However, in the modern day, not many of us are proactive enough to look after our rotator cuffs.

By far, the most common shoulder complaints that I help my clients with are issues involving the rotator cuff. With too much stress or strain over a prolonged period of time, the rotator cuff tendons can degenerate, become painful or even tear. These conditions can be debilitating. A person suffering from rotator cuff problems often struggles to lift their arm, never mind throw a spear. While this isn't as devastating as it would've been in the land of the sabre toothed tiger, it can certainly affect quality of life in the modern world quite dramatically for many.

Rotator cuff problems are also extremely painful, as anyone who's suffered from one will attest to. They are a leading cause of loss of sleep, which only hampers recovery further. And what makes matters worse is that they are bloody difficult to treat!

So, you're far better off avoiding them in the first place if you can help it. One fantastic way of avoiding problems with the rotator cuff is to maintain strength. Strong muscles lead to strong tendons, resistant to shock and the effects of ageing alike[5].

It's very easy to pretend that, because you don't have shoulder pain right now, you're probably fine. Not so. You won't always feel the stress and strain put on the little rotator cuff. In rare cases, people will even experience complete tears of the rotator cuff - imaginatively referred to as 'massive cuff tears' in the medical profession - and not even realise[6]. The problem is, following a massive cuff tear, your shoulder function is now at serious risk.

You don't want to lose the ability to lift your arm over your head. You don't want to risk being unable to throw the ball for your golden retriever, when she's staring at you excitedly with those big, loving eyes.

Far better to take out an insurance policy on one of the most important joints in your body, starting from today. All you need is five minutes every other day, and a can of baked beans to get started.

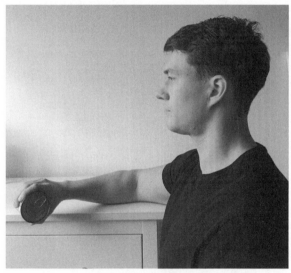

Start sitting next to a table with the elbow of your affected arm resting on the table. Hold a small weight or tin of beans in your hand. Your elbow should be bent to 90 degrees where it will remain throughout.

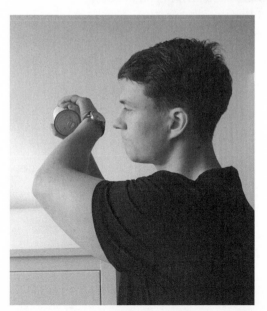

Using your good hand to assist, lift your hand up towards you while still maintaining the 90 degree angle at your elbow. This means that the shoulder is the joint that moves, not the elbow. You may feel a rotating movement occurring at your shoulder joint.

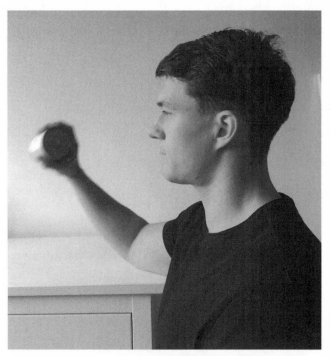

Let go with your good hand and slowly follow the same movement pattern to return the weight to the starting position, to the count of 4-6 seconds. You should feel the muscles around the shoulder having to work to perform this action. When you get to the start position, repeat this exercise up to 10 times, for 3-4 sets. If you don't feel any working ache around the shoulder after 10 repetitions, find something heavier to hold on to.

Getting to Grips with a Painful Shoulder

I frequently see people who have strained their shoulder after a particularly vigorous day of DIY, asking what they should do to get the problem better.

The problem is that it now *really* hurts to lift their arm. Almost all of the exercises you find online for shoulder pain involve raising the arm up overhead. And it's very easy to flare up the symptoms of a shoulder problem, leading to lingering pain for the remainder of the day.

We know that exercises are very important when restoring shoulder health after an injury, but what is one supposed to do when every exercise seems to only worsen the pain?

Do you just push through it? Or do you avoid all of them?

Luckily, there exists an alternative that can grant you relief from your shoulder pain, as well as starting the rehabilitation process. If you've injured the rotator cuff that we spoke about in the previous pages of this book, this simple exercise will prompt the body to start laying down new tissue and begin the healing process. And the best part is that it doesn't even involve moving your arm.

For this exercise, all you're going to do is work on your grip strength. Yes, I realise that you're suffering right now with a shoulder problem, not a hand problem - but hold on a second. Recent research has shown an incredibly strong link between the muscles of the rotator cuff and the muscles we use to grip tightly[7]. Put simply, when the hand grips, the shoulder switches on.

So, to get the crucial muscles of the rotator cuff to start working without suffering the painful process of lifting your arm, all you need to do is grab hold of a sponge or stress ball and start gripping.

I would recommend alternating between gripping and releasing, first very quickly (holding on for just 1 second before relaxing your fingers), and then gripping and squeezing for a longer period of time (holding the contraction for between 5 and 10 seconds). Try doing a couple of minutes of work at each tempo, then see how this affects your shoulder pain after a couple of weeks.

Of course, once your shoulder starts to feel better, you will need to start lifting your arm over your head again to encourage it to heal fully. If you don't eventually get the arm moving again, it will get so stiff that you'll start to lose the ability to perform this action altogether.

However, for the times when it hurts just a little too much to face lifting your arm, you'll always have your gripping exercises to fall back on to awaken the cuff and accelerate the healing process without the sometimes painful side effects of more active exercises.

How to Release a Trapped Nerve

Anyone who's suffered from a trapped nerve in their neck or shoulder knows just how painful it can be. The discomfort can often be felt not only in the area that the nerve is trapped but also down the length of the entire nerve. This can lead to your whole arm becoming painful, not just the problematic area.

This is your body's way of telling you that there's a problem. Symptoms of a trapped nerve can range from pain in the neck, shoulder and arm, to numbness in the hands or even a loss of strength in the limbs. For the purpose of this book, we're only going to talk about trapped nerves that cause pain alone. Any trapped nerve that's giving you pins and needles, numbness or weakness should be assessed by a qualified professional as soon as possible.

A trapped nerve can be caused by a number of different problems in the neck, shoulder or arm. No matter where the root cause of the problem is, the discomfort can be equally unpleasant.

One of the keys to releasing a trapped nerve that I often use with my clients is to gently move the affected limb in a pain-free way as often as possible. Nine times out of ten, the trapped nerve WILL become free - but this process can feel like it takes a very long time to come about, especially when you're in pain! I'd always recommend an assessment from your doctor or a qualified physiotherapist if your nerve pain hasn't subsided after a few weeks.

Here are some tips you can use for relief while you wait for your body to heal and for that trapped nerve to at last become free:

• **Use ice on the most painful areas:** Apply a cold compress, or ice wrapped in a towel, to the painful parts of your arm or shoulder. The ice won't *fix* the problem, but it is nature's pain killer - it dulls the painful nerve transmissions and can bring significant relief. Go for a maximum of 15-minutes each time you use the ice and let the skin heat up to a natural temperature before re-applying. Be careful with any weak or broken skin.

• **Use heat on the neck:** Applying a warm compress or hot water bottle (ensuring you protect your skin) to the neck can help to release any tight muscles in your neck that may be compressing a nerve. By relaxing tight neck muscles, you can encourage the stiff joints beneath to loosen up. Sometimes, this can free a trapped nerve and significantly reduce symptoms. Again, 15-minutes at a time is plenty. In terms of whether to choose ice or heat, it ultimately comes down to personal preference. I recommend starting with ice on the arm (if you have arm pain) and heat on the neck.

• **Use pillows:** If you can feel pain from a trapped nerve when you're sitting in a chair, try placing a stack of firm pillows under the arm of the affected side. I often recommend that my patients place pillows under their arm until their elbow is in line with their armpit (with the arm slightly out to the side). This has the effect of lifting the entire shoulder girdle and relieving the pressure from the nerves around the armpit (which is where the nerves in the arm pass through to reach their final destination). This method can provide comfort when sitting, but don't use it for weeks on end: it can lead to tightness in the neck and shoulder muscles if used too frequently.

- **Sleep positions:** You'll want to avoid sleeping on your front as this necessitates you having to turn your head to the extreme, right or left; not so good for trapped nerves. If you like to sleep on your side, try to place pillows under your head so your head is comfortably in line with your shoulders, not dropped down to one side or propped up too high. If you prefer to sleep on your back, you might want to consider investing in a pillow that has an in-built support that sits in the crook of your neck, maintaining the natural curve of your neck as you rest. These pillows are more and more readily available now from all big retailers - search for an "orthopaedic neck pillow" to find a good selection.

- **Try a change:** I've had patients with neck, shoulder and arm symptoms that I just couldn't figure out. And more times than I can count, eventually, they've come back to me all smiles, saying they suddenly got better. When I enquired why, it becomes clear it had nothing to do with my treatment. *"I just changed the chair I sit in every night and it went away all of a sudden!"* I've heard this more than once; which is why I always recommend to my patients that they experiment with a different chair, a different position of their car seat, even a different bed, and just see how it affects their painful problem. It could well be that the simplest fix for your problem is right under your nose.

CHAPTER THREE

Wrists, Elbows & Hands

Introduction

What sets us apart from the rest of the animal kingdom, other than our superior brain power? I would argue that one of the biggest differences between us and our closest relatives in the natural world is the dexterity and effectiveness with which we are able to use our hands.

Being able to use our hands for intricate, complicated tasks is a huge asset to us as humans. But like any complex process in the body, there are things that can go wrong.

In this chapter, we talk about how to stave off problems with the wrists, elbows and hands for over-fifties, ensuring you remain dextrous and capable as the years pass. We'll talk about how to ward off carpal tunnel syndrome, what tennis elbow really is, and how to ensure your hands stay strong and useful in the garden.

Use those fingers to turn the pages of this chapter and be sure to heed the advice on protecting two of your most valuable assets.

The "Dreaded" Carpal Tunnel Syndrome

Numbness in one hand? Pain around the wrist, thumb and first two or three fingers? It could be carpal tunnel syndrome. A common overuse injury for over-fifties, carpal tunnel syndrome is particularly prevalent in office workers and people who spend a lot of time typing or using a mouse.

As with any numbness, it's important to be checked out by a doctor as soon as possible. However, if you've got a diagnosis of carpal tunnel syndrome, it doesn't necessarily mean you're destined for surgery.

We often see people with carpal tunnel syndrome in our clinic, and most times, we can help them get back to work without needing to go under the knife. But first, it's important to understand what causes carpal tunnel syndrome before we can do something about it.

The "*carpal tunnel*" is a narrow space in the wrist between your carpal bones where a number of tendons (rope-like structures that join muscle to bone), blood vessels and nerves run through. One particular nerve, called the "*median nerve*", is at risk of getting compressed and irritated in the carpal tunnel by the tendons that live so near to it. The median nerve provides sensation and function to your thumb and first two fingers (as well as half of your ring finger), which is why you might be suffering from numbness and pain in these parts of your hand.

Through using the hands and wrist muscles in a repetitive way, some unlucky people find that the tendons in the wrist "rub" on the median nerve. This can irritate, inflame and entrap the nerve, causing the classic symptoms of carpal tunnel syndrome. Luckily, there are ways we can reduce this irritation and help to "free up" that poor nerve in your wrist.

The best thing you can do is, first of all, to try as best as you can to avoid everything that aggravates the problem. This doesn't necessarily mean you need to take time away from the computer; it just means we have to change a few things in your workspace.

The main things to look at are your sitting position, your equipment and your schedule.

You might want to start by experimenting with different chair heights. I know many people undergo an 'ergonomic assessment' with their occupational health department when joining a large company. However, these assessments are primarily designed to help with back and neck pain, and if your last assessment was a long time ago, circumstances may have changed. You might want to adjust your chair and see how that affects your hand and wrist. You might want to move either closer to or further away from your mouse, or bring your computer further towards you, if only temporarily.

The second thing you'll want to look at is the equipment you regularly use. Do you use a standard mouse? Try a vertical mouse instead. Do you use a laptop keyboard? Try a gel pillow that supports your wrist as you type. For those of you who like to sit while you do arts and crafts: is your equipment old or outdated? Try updating it and see how that affects your symptoms.

The third thing to address is your schedule. I don't mean you need to change your working hours; instead, look at your work pattern on a smaller scale. Break your work up into half-hour chunks. When you've finished your half an hour, take two minutes to stand up, stretch and rest your hands. Adding in regular micro-breaks can help stave off the symptoms of carpal tunnel syndrome and other upper limb conditions[1].

Once you've addressed these things in your workplace or at home, you may want to look at relieving some of the tension in your wrist through a selection of gentle stretches. The tendons that irritate the median nerve belong to a set of muscles called the "wrist flexors". If you bend your wrist so as to try and touch your forearm with the fingers of the same hand, you can see and feel your wrist flexors at work on the inside of your forearm.

When the wrist flexors become tight, the symptoms of carpal tunnel syndrome are more likely. So, it would make sense that stretching these muscles to lengthen them slightly can help to relieve symptoms.

Stop the stretch if it makes your symptoms worse and get checked by a doctor for suitability before commencing with this stretching programme.

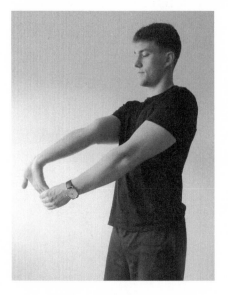

Straighten the arm to be stretched and lift it in front of you with the palm facing up. Using your other hand, pull the fingers and wrist gently back as shown until you feel a stretch in the forearm of the painful side. Hold this gentle stretch for 30-seconds x 4-5 per day.

The Truth About Tennis Elbow

Tennis elbow? That's just for professional tennis players, right?

Actually, tennis elbow is one of the most common conditions I am asked about by people of all ages in my clinic. And guess what? *Almost none of the sufferers play tennis!*

Tennis elbow is characterised by a painful area around the bone on the outside of your elbow. It might be sore to touch and it is likely to feel worse whenever you grip firmly or lift something heavy.

Now, there is something that almost always surprises my patients about tennis elbow. And that is that tennis elbow is *absolutely nothing* to do with the elbow joint at all!

Let me explain…

Even though the pain you *feel* with tennis elbow is right on the elbow bone, the *problem* is somewhere else entirely. The real problem is actually in your **wrist**.

The muscles that control your wrist live in your forearm. They control the wrist by pulling on long tendons that run into the hand, allowing you to open jars, control a steering wheel and turn the pages of this book. These muscles live in the forearm, but some of them attach to one of the bones on the side of your elbow via a short tendon. This tendon connects to the area that is painful with tennis elbow.

Tennis elbow is actually a problem with this small tendon; so, even though the problematic tendon is close to the elbow, it actually has no control over the elbow joint at all - the tendon and the muscle attached to it controls the *wrist* instead!

Tennis elbow is categorised as an **overuse injury of the wrist, not the elbow**. It is common in people who do a lot of DIY; think about the action of turning a screwdriver over and over and over again. This kind of job involves a lot of wrist work, but not much effort from the elbow.

So, now we know a bit about tennis elbow, what can we do to help it?

With any overuse injury, there is a fundamental mis-match between the amount of work you're trying to do and the strength of the muscles trying to perform the work.

Think about it this way: if you started training for a marathon and gradually built up from running half a mile to a full 26.2 miles over the course of two years, your muscles would likely be strong enough to cope with the demands you're asking of them. However, if you got up off the couch today and decided to run 26.2 miles right off the bat, how do you think your body would respond?

It wouldn't like it! Not one bit.

And the same is often true for people who develop tennis elbow. They go from not using their wrists very much, to suddenly using a screw driver for four hours at a time trying to build that new flat pack wardrobe.

If this kind of thing has happened to you, you're certainly not alone (I've done it myself plenty of times, despite knowing better)! You're also not necessarily going to be stuck with this painful elbow either - below, I'll show you a method I use with my clients to help them recover from tennis elbow.

Use the exercise below to strengthen your wrist muscles and recover from tennis elbow. It's a good idea to lay off the DIY for a few weeks, too! However, you *can* eventually get back to building that wardrobe (or that yearly tennis game) soon - just wait until the pain has resolved first!

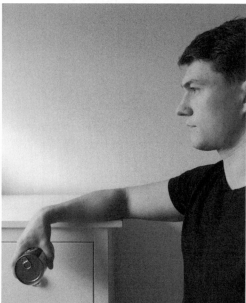

Start with your affected arm supported on a table. The forearm does not move position throughout the entire exercise. Hold something with a modest weight in your hand, i.e. a small dumbbell or a tin of beans. Start with the weight hanging down as shown.

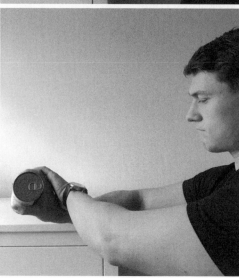

Use your good hand to assist your painful hand by pulling the weight upwards, bringing your knuckles towards you. The forearm or elbow does not move, only the wrist.

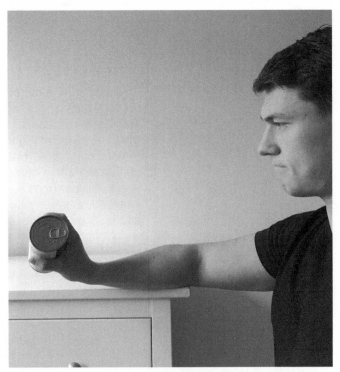

Let go with your good hand and very slowly control the weight back to the starting position, to the count of 4 or 5 seconds. The muscles working here are the wrist muscles that control the forearm. When you get back to the start position, repeat the exercise up to 10 times, every few hours throughout the day. If you can do more than 10 repetitions before getting a working ache in your forearm, find something heavier to hold.

The Truth About Golfer's Elbow

Golfer's elbow is very similar to tennis elbow. This condition causes a painful point in your elbow too, except on the other side of the joint (the bony point closest to your side when your arm is hanging down; below).

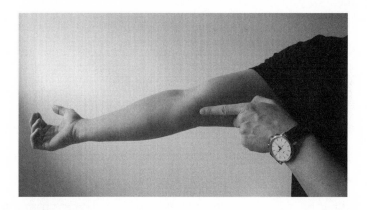

Just like tennis elbow, this problem often starts after some DIY or a long day of sport of some kind (however, I have yet to treat anyone suffering from this injury as a genuine result of golf!)

Golfer's elbow, just like tennis elbow, is also caused by a problem with the tendons of your wrist muscles, not your elbow. If you put your hand out in front of you as if you were holding a plate of food, then try to touch the inside of your wrist with your fingers, you'll be using a group of muscles called your 'wrist flexors'. It is these muscles that are at the root of the problem in golfer's elbow.

Golfer's elbow is a repetitive strain injury, causing a problem with the tendon that joins these muscles to the bone. Because the tendon attaches the muscle to a bone in the elbow, the pain experienced in this condition is felt in your elbow.

One common story I often hear is of a client of mine going to play badminton, deciding to play for half an hour longer than they normally would, then developing a very tender point on their inner elbow. This is the early stage of golfer's elbow!

Luckily, for most people, they rest the arm for a day or two and the problem disappears, never to be seen again. However, for some unlucky people, golfer's elbow can persist far beyond a few days. This is particularly the case for someone whose job involves lots of repetitive hand and wrist movements - giving the tendon no chance to recover.

It also unfortunately occurs for many people who decide to get into resistance training in their advancing age. Despite this, I always recommend people over fifty start some kind of resistance training programme (if their health allows), as the benefits are simply too great to ignore. As Arnold Schwarzenneger allegedly once said, *"Are you too old to lift weights? You are too old NOT to lift weights!"*

That being said, unfortunately the repetitive pulling motion involved with a lot of weight training exercises can set off this kind of elbow pain and become troublesome for a lot of people. If you're just starting out a new hobby and have developed this elbow pain, it can really put a dampener on things.

But fear not! There are a few steps you can put into action to reverse the problem and have that elbow feeling a bit better soon:

 • **If you've just developed some elbow pain, it's a good idea to take 3 days' rest from the activity that caused it in the first place.** For many people, this will be enough to resolve the pain.

• **Right after the pain starts, it's a good idea to put ice on the painful area** (be sure to protect the skin). Although there isn't usually a huge amount of *inflammation* present in golfer's elbow, there might be some swelling present in the first few days of the condition. Icing the area for 15 minutes at a time will help to control this, minimising the pain and any inflammation.

• **You could consider an elbow support.** While this won't fix the condition, it will provide support to the joint and can limit further sprains and strains with a painful elbow if you have some unavoidable DIY to finish off.

• **To fix the condition, we need to take the same approach as with tennis elbow** (on the previous pages), just with a slightly different exercise in terms of your wrist positioning. We need to strengthen the wrist muscles so they can meet the demands you're asking of them. As the muscles involved here are different, you're going to need a different exercise. If your doctor is happy for you to try the exercise on the following page, go ahead and give it a go:

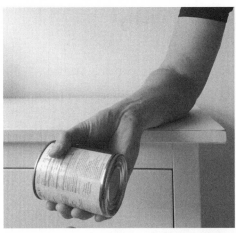

Start holding onto something with a small weight in your affected hand, such as a light dumbbell or tin of beans. Rest your forearm on a table with the palm up and wrist relaxed, as shown in the picture.

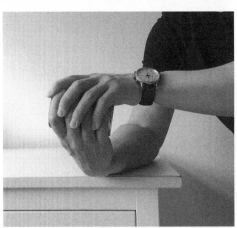

Using your good hand to assist the movement, bring your fingers and the weight up towards you, moving only the wrist - NOT the elbow. Your forearm must remain in contact with the table at all times, as shown.

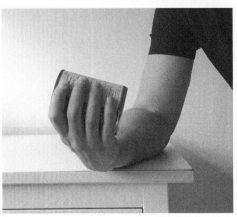

Then let go with your good hand and return to the start position in a slow, controlled manner, to the count of 4 or 5 seconds. When you get to the start position, repeat up to 10 times, every few hours throughout the day. If you can do more than 10 repetitions before you get a working ache in your forearm, find something heavier to hold.

Don't Lose Your Grip!

For those reading this who are fifty or older, I've got some bad news for you: every year, you're going to lose roughly 1% of your muscle mass as you go through the ageing process[2].

Sadly, this is just a fact of life and you're not alone; it's happening to your friends too. The problem is, this loss of muscle mass isn't just cosmetic; it leads to a loss of strength as well[3]. This loss of strength is often the driver behind many common physical problems.

Busy people like you and I use a lot of strength each day without even realising. Climbing stairs, carrying bags and walking the dog every day all require significant use of the muscles throughout our bodies. The parts of our body that we use arguably more than anything else are our hands - and they are no different when it comes to the ageing process.

Our hands allow us to secure a tight grip around heavy objects, as well as perform delicate, dextrous tasks, such as doing up buttons or writing a letter. Our hands separate us from the rest of the animal kingdom. The sheer versatility of our hands means it's our duty to take care of them.

Our hands suffer with a loss of muscle mass as much as our larger muscles do. Without sufficient strength in your hands, life becomes far more difficult. For this reason, it is worth taking out a figurative "insurance policy" on these fantastic tools! You can do this, and thereby resist the process of ageing, by strengthening your grip in times of quiet and relaxation. By doing this, you can be confident that your hands won't let you down in more urgent circumstances when you need them most.

There are two ways of strengthening the grip that I like to share with my clients. The first way is to practice the action of repetitive gripping and relaxing, squeezing your fingers hard into a sponge, as fast as you can. This helps to work the muscle to fatigue and may help to lubricate the joints in the fingers as well, protecting against arthritis.

The second way is to grip the sponge as hard as you can, then squeeze for a duration of 10-seconds. This method helps you prepare for the long walk from the shops to the car while holding bags housing the entirety of the Christmas shopping. This type of exercise involves the muscles having to contract as hard as they can for a sustained period of time.

All you'll need for these exercises is a sponge or a soft, squeezy ball. If you've got known arthritis in your hands, here's a top tip: run a basin full of warm water and plunge your hands into it while doing the exercises - it'll help loosen those stiff finger joints.

The pictures below will show you the exercises that I share with my clients to improve their grip and maintain the health of their most important tools:

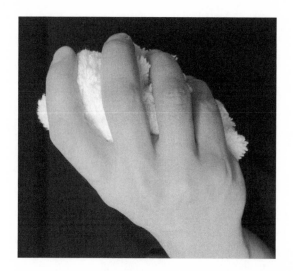

This gripping exercise can be done in two ways:
1. Gripping the sponge and relaxing as quickly as you can for 30-seconds at a time.
2. Gripping the sponge and squeezing as tight as you can for 10-seconds, then repeating 3 times over.

Both of these methods are effective and should be performed in sets of 3-4 per day.

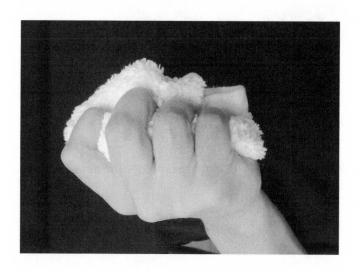

Rescue Arthritic Thumbs

Pain in the thumb-side of your hand? Difficulty gripping anything between your thumb and your forefinger? It's possible that you could be suffering with the early signs of thumb arthritis.

Arthritis of the thumb usually appears at one of the joints in the hand that most people don't realise exists. You can see a picture below showing the most common joint that thumb arthritis affects:

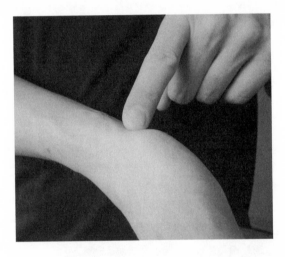

Now, many people will tell you that once you've started to develop arthritis in your thumbs, it's all downhill from here and maybe that you'll soon lose the use of your grip altogether. The truth is, for most people, this really isn't the case!

Provided it is caught and treated early, there are plenty of things you can do to relieve some of the pain associated with thumb arthritis and possibly limit how much further it advances. I've had to personally read up on ways of looking after my own thumbs so I can continue to practice as a physiotherapist for years to come. Coming from a professional football background, my treatment style is very "hands-on"; this certainly takes a toll on your hands and thumbs, as you can probably imagine!

If you've got arthritic thumbs, you may notice "nodules" appearing around the small joints in your thumb. They often give the joints in the thumb the appearance that they are "bigger" than they were before. These nodules appear because the body has started to lay down extra bone around the joint in an attempt to spread any load that you are putting through your thumb. It's yet another way that the body is extremely clever and sophisticated in the way it tries to manage stress and strain. However, these nodules can be unpleasant to look at and are a cause of great concern for many people that I speak to. Unfortunately, at the time of writing there aren't any known ways for reducing them in size or stop them from forming.

You may also find that the pain isn't necessarily in your thumb, but more in your hand and wrist, on the thumb side. This is because we have a "hidden" thumb joint that sits closer to the wrist than it does to the palm of the hand. It is this joint that seems to be affected most commonly by arthritis, as you can see in the picture above.

If you're suffering from stiffness and pain in your thumb or in the thumb side of the hand, here are some things that may help it:

• **Try using heat:** Applying a hot water bottle to the sore area in the morning and evening (being careful to protect the skin) can help to relieve tension in the hand and improve circulation in the affected area.

Heat can also help to loosen up stiff joints so that you can move your hand a bit better, especially in the first 15 minutes after you wake up.

• **Grab a sponge and run a basin full of warm water:** I like to give this tip to many of my clients with thumb arthritis. I often tell them to fill a basin with warm water and plunge a sponge into it. They can then exercise the affected thumb by pressing the thumb into the sponge (as if squeezing it between thumb and palm) while submerged in the water. This helps in two ways; first, you get the positive effects of the warm water which helps to lubricate movement. Second, you get the strengthening effect of using the muscles around the thumb. This helps you to better cope with the demands of your day-to-day use of that thumb as it should be stronger and more capable than it was before. This usually leads to less pain, too. Bear in mind that it can take up to 12 weeks before any significant strength is gained anywhere in the body, and this applies to your thumb too.

• **In the cold, make sure you wear your gloves:** When you're suffering from thumb arthritis, one of the worst things you can do is to let your hands get cold. Because our hands are an extremity, the blood from this part of our body tends to rush toward our middle whenever we get cold. This is because the body recognises that the heart and other organs are the most important asset we have, so it sacrifices blood flow to the hands to protect our key organs. This means that, as soon as the cold weather creeps in, our hands suffer worst! By remembering to take a pair of warm gloves with you in the car or in your coat pocket, you can protect against the chills and avoid the stiffness and pain that having cold hands can bring.

CHAPTER FOUR

Back Pain & Sciatica

Introduction

Eighty percent of us will suffer from back pain at some point in our lives, whether it be for a day, a month or several years[1]. How we manage back pain is still a fiercely debated topic in modern medicine; it is the leading cause of physical disability worldwide and is responsible for an enormous share of work absences each year.

Despite the back pain epidemic, we still don't fully understand all the nuances of back pain. It may still be one of science's most challenging modern mysteries, never having been conclusively cracked or solved, despite some progress in recent years.

It is only right, seeing as I help people with back problems more than anything else, that I include a chapter about back pain (and its close relative, sciatica) in this book. My aim with this chapter is to teach you a bit about what we *do* know about this problem, as well as giving you some of the tools to help and prevent it, should you wish to apply my lessons.

Leave your expectations and current beliefs at the door for this one; some of the following facts and methods may surprise you... but don't let that put you off! Read on to learn the truth about back pain, how the body is more interconnected than you might think, as well as some simple methods that are proven to help stop back pain in its tracks.

The Truth About Back Pain

Through millennia of pain and suffering, as humans, we have been conditioned to associate *pain* with *damage* - both physically and emotionally.

As children, when we cut our hand on the shard of glass we tried to pick up to show Mum, we felt the sharp pain and saw the bleeding from our finger. When we ran too fast in the playground and fell, breaking our arm or grazing our knees, we felt the pain associated with the damage that we've caused our bodies.

These experiences stick with us forever. Most of the time, our experiences ring true - when we damage our bodies, we experience pain.

However, there are also times when the pain we experience and the physical damage that has actually occurred to our body *fails* to match up. And when these situations occur, it runs counter to everything we've experienced as developing children.

Take back pain, for instance. For many years, we assumed that back pain was caused solely by damage to one of a number of structures within the spine. Twenty years ago, if someone came to us with back pain, we would tell them they had pulled a muscle, sprained a joint or damaged a disc. We would say that the pain would be there for as long as the tissue was injured, and when the injury heals, the pain will resolve.

We now know that this theory is flawed. Over many years of medical study, and the brilliant research into pain done by scientists and clinicians alike, we now know that it is possible, and very common in fact, for people to experience pain in the complete absence of physical injury[2].

This means that if you've suffered from back, neck or shoulder pain at any time in your life, there's actually a good chance that there was no physical damage occurring whatsoever in that area, despite all the painful clues suggesting otherwise.

Although relevant to any part of the body, I have included this chapter in the "*Back Pain*" section of this book because it seems that experiencing pain in the absence of true injury is one of the most common causes of back pain in the people I see in my clinic. It is a phenomenon I witness firsthand every single day.

I recently saw a patient who had been suffering with back pain for the last nine months. She'd finally got fed up, and had paid out of pocket for an MRI scan.

She got her MRI scan results a week later. *"The report says there's NOTHING wrong with my back... But the pain is still there! They must have read the pictures wrong. I **know** what I feel,"* she lamented to me directly after.

But the truth is, the doctors didn't read the pictures wrong at all. What my patient didn't yet understand was that although there was no *physical* injury to her back, it didn't mean that she wasn't telling the truth, nor that her pain was insignificant. A scan can show damaged structures, but it cannot show movement problems, muscle weakness, tightness or joint stiffness. After an assessment, I could quickly identify the problem.

When I asked my patient to bend forward and try to touch her toes, the problem was obvious. She was hardly able to move her spine at all! She was able to reach for the floor... But all of her available movement was coming from her hips.

With a few small tweaks to her movement, some targeted stretches and some practice at home, my patient was able to resolve her back pain within eight weeks of us first meeting.

Now, let me ask you a question:

Did you wake up one day with a nagging ache in your lower back? Did it progressively worsen, despite you not remembering a clear incident that could've injured your back? This is a story I hear all the time. The truth about this kind of back pain is that usually there isn't a strain or a sprain or a trapped nerve causing the pain. This is the same story that my patient came to me with.

In situations like this, back pain can be caused by a combination of tightness in some areas, weakness in others, problems with movement patterns and even changes to the way your brain is processing signals from that area of the body. As you can see from all that you've just read, it's entirely possible that your back pain is far more complex than you might have originally thought.

But don't despair! There are some positives we can take from all this. Firstly, back pain caused by muscle tightness, weakness and movement problems can be solved without needing to go under the surgeon's knife. As a physiotherapist, I've built a career around this fact!

We now know that opting to have surgery because of back pain before trying anything else can be one of the worst things you can do. It can even make the problem worse[3]. For this reason, we only recommend surgery as a last resort.

Secondly, because of the fact that back pain often isn't caused by physical damage to your back, it might be the case that getting an MRI scan would be a complete waste of your time and money.

We can't *see* back pain on a scan. But quite often, we will see lots and lots of age-related changes on the results of a scan, even in pain-free people[4], and especially for those over fifty. What this means is that it's down to the best guess of your doctor as to what structure in that MRI picture is responsible for your pain. Put simply, it's impossible for us to accurately tell if it's the issue seen on the scan that is causing your pain, or something else entirely.

The other problem is that pain can move around. We don't necessarily feel pain directly in the problem area. I've had patients who came to see me about their knee pain… but the problem was actually their hip joint! The same is true for your back.

There are situations where an MRI scan is a good idea. These situations are beyond the scope of this book. This is one reason why it's important to speak to your doctor or physiotherapist first about any new onset of back pain; they can tell you whether or not a scan is appropriate for you.

I hope this section has answered more questions about back pain than it has raised! It's important to remember that 99% of back pain is "non-serious" - that is, it won't kill you and it is treatable.

As always, get any new case of back pain checked out, but try not to worry! It's likely that you haven't damaged anything. You might just need a helping hand in getting better.

How Your Back Can Cause Pain In Your Leg

Have you ever heard of the term "*sciatica*"?

Lots of people have heard of sciatica; maybe their friend suffered from it, or they've read something about it online. However, unless they've suffered from it themselves and been forced to learn a bit more, few people actually understand what sciatica is or how it comes about.

Sciatica is a term used to describe pain in the leg related to the sciatic nerve.

The sciatic nerve is the longest, thickest nerve in the human body. It starts in the lower back and runs all the way down the back of the leg to the toes. You have one sciatic nerve in each leg, and it's roughly an inch in diameter at its widest point.

The sciatic nerve is very important. It allows us to use our legs to walk, as well as feel sensation in our feet. But when it's trapped, irritated or pinched, it can produce immense pain that runs all the way down the back of the leg into the foot. It can also cause pins and needles and numbness in the feet - a symptom that can be very alarming.

So, what causes this nerve to get trapped or irritated?

Usually, the problem actually occurs within a person's lower back. When the sciatic nerve branches off from the spinal cord to run down the leg, it must pass through some very tight spaces between the bones and discs in your back.

If there's a problem with one of the joints or discs in your lower back, the nerve can get pinched in the tight spaces it usually travels through quite happily. This causes sciatica - and as anyone who's suffered from this problem before can attest to, it is incredibly painful!

Another place the nerve can get trapped or irritated is in your bottom. Did you know that we put pressure on the sciatic nerve every time we sit on a chair or the toilet? You can test this out yourself by sitting on the toilet for a prolonged period of time and seeing what happens; I'll bet you end up with pins and needles in your feet when you stand up again! That's the sciatic nerve being compressed by the hard toilet seat.

Usually, we can cope with a bit of pressure on the sciatic nerve. But if we have tight bottom muscles, the sciatic nerve can get trapped here too.

It's very difficult for you to self-diagnose where your sciatica is coming from and I wouldn't recommend trying. That's why it's important to be looked at by a doctor or physiotherapist who can work out where the problem is coming from and make a plan to treat it.

As we move through this book, you'll likely come across lots of examples of problems in the body that aren't as they seem; not least, a back problem causing pain or numbness in your toes.

If these concepts seem confusing, don't be concerned! The human body is very complex and we're still trying to fully understand certain aspects of it. The main thing to remember is that the more you're aware of how these problems can arise, the better prepared you'll be to avoid and remedy them if you do start to suffer at some point in the future.

Now, let's talk about a novel way of relieving sciatica that I've found very effective in the past for many of my clients.

My Approach to Stretching for Sciatica Relief

Through my work as a physiotherapist in my clinic, I have become known as a specialist in helping people with back problems and sciatica.

One of the reasons I have had more success than most when it comes to sciatica is the fact that my approach is very different to the approaches you might find online, or in your average clinic.

Once I've assessed my patient and decided that nothing "sinister" is causing their sciatica (this may involve getting MRI scans done prior to treatment in some cases), I tell most people to disregard the typical stretches they've seen online claiming to be the "best" exercises for sciatica.

Why? Because these exercises are largely ineffective for most of the people I help!

If you look online, the typical approach towards exercises for sciatica begins by stretching the muscles in the affected leg.The problem with this approach is that it often makes people WORSE, not better!

The reason for this, I believe, is the following fact: Nerves absolutely hate to be stretched![5]

When you stretch a nerve, you aggravate the area which can cause inflammation to increase in many cases. Unfortunately, most of the stretches recommended for sciatica don't just stretch the muscles in the leg… They stretch the sciatic nerve too!

In this way, in the process of doing something good (stretching the muscles), we inadvertently do something bad (stretch the nerve). This leads to either no change, or to the symptoms getting worse. Either way, the result is not good for the poor person who diligently went online to search for a way to fix their problem.

This is another reason why I tell my clients not to rely on YouTube videos for the most-part - it is possible to make the problem worse much of the time!

Luckily, I've found a far more effective way of helping people with sciatica. It's not perfect and it isn't effective every time, but it works more than the usual approach from my experience in clinic.

Here's the approach; it's very simple. I focus my client's exercises around stretching the NON-painful leg… whilst leaving the painful leg well alone.

I know this an unusual concept, but there's some recent evidence to support my theory[6]. The human body is very clever and we're starting to see proof of the fact that when you make a change on the left side of your body, in some circumstances a similar change happens on the right side too.

When we're in pain, certain parts of our body work to compensate for the areas that aren't working well any longer. This often means that our right side can become tight and restricted even when it's our left leg that's hurting. By stretching the right side (if the left is painful), we can often indirectly help the left leg.

This approach also means that we avoid aggravating the painful leg and everything calms down as a result.

Before I share two of the exercises I commonly use with you, it's important to note that these exercises aren't suitable for everyone and there's no way for me to tell if they'll help you or not. That's why it's vital you get checked out by your doctor or physiotherapist before putting these exercises into action.

That being said, let's have a look at two of the common ones I recommend my clients with this issue:

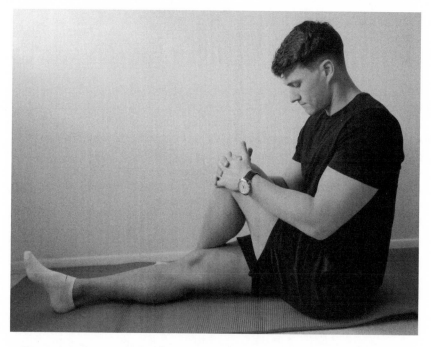

Start sitting on the floor (either unsupported as shown or with a wall at your back for comfort). Fold the leg to be stretched (the non-painful side) over the other leg and plant the foot on the floor. Grab the knee with both hands and pull towards your opposite shoulder until you feel a stretch in your buttock (on the non-painful side). Hold for 30-seconds and repeat 4-5 times.

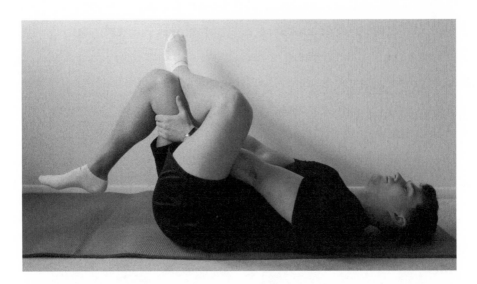

In this picture, the left leg is the one being stretched. You are going to stretch your non-painful side for this exercise. Lying on your back with your knees bent. Cross the non-painful leg over the painful leg so the non-painful shin is in contact with your opposite thigh. Reach through the gap between your legs and pull your painful leg gently up towards you as shown in the picture. This will lift the non-painful leg into a stretch which targets the gluteal muscles and the piriformis muscle. Hold for 30-seconds, repeating 5 times each day.

How Sitting Affects Your Back

It's no secret that working an office job where you sit in a chair for eight hours, five days a week, forty eight weeks of the year, has the potential to place you at risk of having a bad back[7].

But why is this the case?

Surely people who keep their backs immobilised for most of the day avoid "wear and tear" or "sprains and strains" far better than more active workers?

Well, that is true to some extent. However, every job has its own unique profile of health risks. Sitting for much of our lives has a different, more insidious effect on our backs[8].

For a start, in the absence of long bouts of exercise done regularly before or after work, sitting for long periods of time, day after day, causes you to lose a lot of the muscle strength in your back and midriff. This area is referred to collectively as your "*core*". You may have heard of this before if you've ever taken a Pilates class.

The core acts as a sort of corset to keep your spine and midriff stable when you move. It's an important part of your anatomy. Sitting doesn't involve much core stability, so if all we do is sit, our core gets weaker and weaker over time through disuse. This weakness can leave us vulnerable to back trouble as soon as we put any significant stress on the spine, such as when lifting something heavy from the floor.

The other reason that sitting can be bad for our backs comes down to our evolution as humans. We weren't built to sit - we were built to walk, squat and run. When we sit, we're putting lots of muscle groups in our hips and pelvis into a shortened position. Over time, if nothing is done to counter it, this shortened position becomes permanent. This may contribute to the fact that, in one study, almost half of all office workers reported being uncomfortable with their work station at their job[8].

The muscles at the front of our hips, called the "hip flexors", are significantly shortened when we sit. If we sit a lot, they remain tight even when we stand up. This can lead to a "tilt" in the pelvis, as the tight muscles pull the pelvis forward. We call this an "*anterior pelvic tilt*", which is a fancy term to describe the "duck-like" appearance that some people have when they walk around (characterised by bums and tummies sticking out).

This position can put stress on the back when held for a long period of time. It may be one of the most common factors contributing to back pain in office workers[9]. The problem is, this postural change happens so slowly that no one notices. However, try looking at yourself side-on in a mirror; is your bottom sticking out? Are the bony points at the front of your hips tilted forward? If you answered "yes" to either of these questions, you could be suffering with an excessive anterior pelvic tilt.

If you think you might be developing this issue, don't panic! There are a few things you can do to combat the effects of sitting and gradually reverse the postural change you have developed.

Firstly, it's important to try to minimise unnecessary sitting from this point onwards. You can't change your job, but you can minimise the length of time you spend sitting outside of work.

The other alternative is to check out standing desks for your workplace. These desks give you the option of standing up while you work. They represent a great way to break up the 8-hours of sitting we do during a working day.

Secondly, it's important to stretch out the tight areas at the front of the hips to prevent this tightness from building up and tugging the pelvis down or tilting it forwards. There are a couple of simple stretches you can do regularly to counter the effects of sitting. I've included a diagram below showing you one of the best ones:

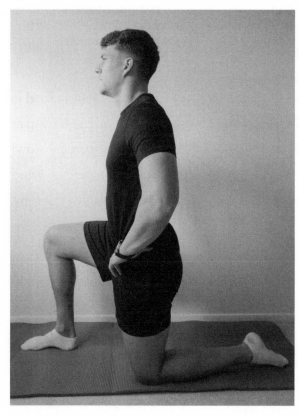

Step 1: Start kneeling on a soft surface. The knee that is in contact with the ground is the side that is going to be stretched.

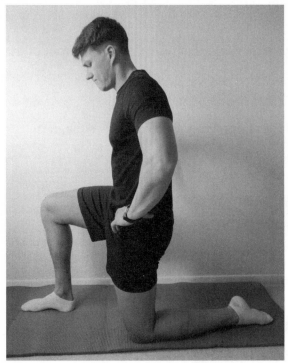

Step 2: Imagine you are trying to tuck your tailbone underneath you, as you rotate your pelvis and squeeze your buttocks together. You should feel a stretch at the front of the thigh (in this picture the left side is being stretched). Hold this stretch for 30-seconds and repeat 4-5 times on each side, each day.

Control Your Core

Once the interest of just gymnasts and martial artists, the concept of "core strengthening" has sky-rocketed in popularity over the last ten years or so, in part due to the rise of Pilates.

Pilates is an approach to exercise often taught in classes. It mainly involves attempting to use the tummy muscles (collectively referred to as "the core") to control the midriff and spine during certain movements. The goal of this exercise approach is to provide a stable base, from which you can move your limbs safely with a lowered risk of injury[10].

While core training isn't the be-all and end-all in terms of injury prevention (as some practitioners would have you believe), having a nice, stable midriff is important.

Think of your core as a strong foundation. The rest of your body (your limbs and spine) are the buildings built on top of that foundation. If we have a weak, unstable foundation, how do you think the buildings on top of it are going to fare? Chances are, not very well.

One of the problems with modern life is that we spend a lot of time in very comfortable positions. Our chairs and car seats tend to support us very well whenever we sit, which means that our tummy muscles get a free ride. This makes them lazy and weak over a period of time. This is not good. Without sufficient strength in your midriff, you cannot maintain safe control of your spine. While this might not be a problem for very basic movements, as soon as we overreach slightly, we are put at heightened risk of injury.

You might've heard a story from a friend or family member where they tried to bend down and twist for something that had fallen on the floor, when suddenly they developed back pain. Many times, this is the sign of a weak core that has failed to do its job - protecting their lower back.

In this way, you can think of the core as the bodyguard of your spine. When it's nice and strong, it minimises the harm that can come to your back when you push slightly too far in a certain direction.

So, how can we prevent the core from becoming weak? And if we are suffering with a weak core, how do we turn things around?

A good first step towards improving things would be to get active! Walking is one great way of making the core work. This week, try to walk slightly further than you normally do by adding in one or two extra fifteen-minute walks over the course of the week, as long as walking is a comfortable activity for you.

The second step of improving your core strength is to work on "switching on" the core muscles. This is a great exercise to practice in bed or at home, providing it isn't painful for you to perform and there are no individual reasons why it isn't suitable for you:

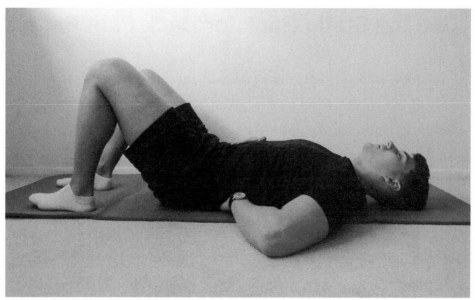

Start lying on your back either on a bed or on the floor with your knees bent half way. Place your hand under the small of your back as shown. You should initially feel that it is easy to place your hand under your back due to the natural curve in your spine. Now, activate your tummy muscles and squeeze your buttocks gently so as to close the gap between your lower back and the floor/bed. You should feel the pressure increase on your hand. Hold this gentle contraction for 10-seconds, then relax, repeating 10 times in a row. Do this regularly throughout the day.

Use the Static Back for Back Pain Relief

As a physiotherapist, my main goal with my clients is to improve their quality of life; this often involves working with clients to restore their mobility, improve their independence and get them back to the things they love. However, one of the other very important things that people ask for when they see me is pain relief.

Back pain can be a particularly tricky issue to overcome because of its unpredictable nature. What helps one person to experience some degree of pain relief only serves to make another feel even worse.

That's another reason why finding exercises to do on YouTube can be a real minefield. It's always best to get exercises customised to your specific needs when it comes to back pain.

That being said, there is a position that I recommend to many of my back pain clients that very often provides some degree of relief. It's a position that was discovered by a leading therapist who invented an approach to treating painful problems called the Egoscue Method™.

The thing I like about this exercise is that it's very simple to do and there's only a small chance it will make symptoms worse. That being said, no exercise is suitable for everyone so be sure to get checked out by a doctor or physiotherapist before putting this one into action. As you'll also see, if you are unable to get down and up again from the floor, this one probably isn't for you.

This exercise is called the "Static Back" and it's simply a position you can get into that takes pressure off the spine. Getting into this position, even just for a few moments each day, can be enough to ease off the symptoms of a stiff and sore back.

The goal of the time spent in this position is to allow your spine to 'flatten' as much as possible into the floor. I usually recommend to my clients that they try to remain in this position for 5 minutes at a time (although many choose to stay there a lot longer - it can be an amazingly comfortable position!)

See below for the proper technique for the Static Back exercise:

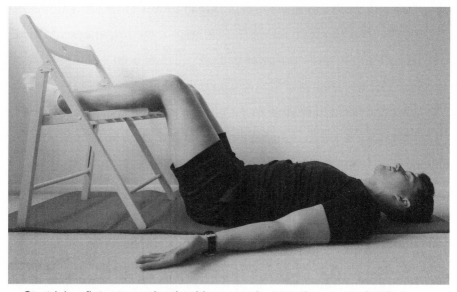

Start lying flat on your back with your calves resting on a raised surface, like a chair. Your knees and hips should be as close to 90 degree angles as possible. Put your hands out to your sides at around a 45 degree angle with the palms facing upwards. Try to relax your spine, section by section, and feel it relaxing into the floor. There should be no effort spent performing in this exercise; it is purely a relaxing position for pain relief.

How Your FEET Can Cause Back Pain

Now, this may surprise you, but your feet could truly be a contributing cause of the pain you may currently suffer in your lower back[11].

Your feet are very important. They are usually the only part of your body that makes contact with the floor. If you think about it, they support the weight of your entire body for many hours each and every day.

This means that if you have a problem with your feet, there's likely to be a knock-on effect all the way up through the weight-bearing joints in the body. The main weight-bearing joints are our ankles, knees and hips, followed by the joints in our lower back. If the feet aren't doing their job properly, somewhere else has to pick up the slack!

So, how can you tell if your feet aren't doing their job properly?

The best way to tell is to be assessed by a professional who's got experience in dealing with bottom-up issues like most foot problems. However, you can also get some clues by looking at your feet yourself.

Go and stand barefoot in front of a full-length mirror and spend some time looking at your feet. What do you see?

Do you have a nice arch in your instep? Or do your feet roll inwards?

Are your toes nice and straight? Or are some of them twisted and squashed together?

Do you have corns, calluses or bunions?

All of these questions can help you determine how "healthy" your feet are. One of the biggest problems we see when assessing the feet of clients in my clinic is, by far, "flat feet". Flat feet is the common expression used to describe the appearance of having no instep arch. This may make the ankle look like it's rolling inwards.

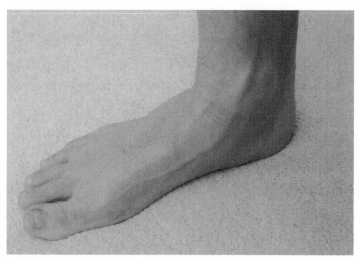

A flat foot: the instep arch has disappeared as the foot has rolled inwards.

The problem with flat feet is that having this issue causes a dramatic change to the way that force is transmitted through the lower limbs into the floor[12]. Instead of the force of our body weight traveling straight down through the legs as it was designed, the force will now move in an angular way through the hips, ankles and knees. This places excess pressure through the joints and can lead to an increase in stress on these areas. In addition to being a potential cause of knee and hip pain, flat feet may also cause back pain in the exact same way.

So, what causes flat feet? One of the most common causes of flat feet is a loss of strength in the tiny muscles we have in our feet. Just like in our arms and hands, we have muscles in our feet too, which help us to control our walking and balance. For a number of reasons, which we'll discuss later, we can lose strength in these small muscles. Flat feet can also be caused by genetic, structural problems that we inherit from our parents.

If you're suffering from flat feet, you may notice aches and pains in your hips, knees and ankles as well as your lower back. But it's also possible that you won't feel any pain at all; some people live with flat feet quite happily their whole lives and never suffer as a result. What this means is that if you've got flat feet and back pain, it isn't necessarily the flat feet *causing* the back pain, but it could be a contributing factor.

If you do have flat feet, the more active you are, the greater your risk of suffering from one of these problems elsewhere in the body that are linked to your feet.

If you think you do have flat feet, here are some things you can try to help:

- **Don't always wear supportive footwear:** While this sounds counterintuitive, wearing supportive shoes all the time can actually CAUSE flat feet. This happens because when we wear comfortable, supportive shoes, they do the job of the tiny muscles in our feet, meaning our foot muscles get a free ride. Because they don't need to work as hard any longer, they switch off and become lazy and weak. This can contribute to the loss of your arch, as your foot muscles aren't strong enough to maintain it any more.

- **However, when you're out for a long walk, it might be an idea to try an arch support:** While I don't believe it is a good idea to wear arch supports or insoles around the house or throughout normal life for most people due to the reasons outlined above, if you know you're heading out for a long walk today, getting an insole that supports the dropped arch can be an effective way of protecting your joints. Insoles are the layers of either fabric or plastic that you can buy from most chemists and put inside your shoe. They help to support weak areas of the foot and temporarily 'fix' a dropped arch. Just be sure not to wear these insoles for too long, despite how good they might feel, as they take over from your important foot muscles and can lead to weakness.

- **Work on lifting your arch when standing or sitting for a few minutes each day:** This is a surprisingly challenging thing to do. While sitting or standing, try to lift the inner part of your foot by using your foot muscles, without letting your toes or heel lift from the floor. You might feel as though your foot is going to cramp up when you first start practicing this, but over a period of several months your feet will get stronger and be better able to support your weight without the arch 'collapsing'. This exercise has been shown to be effective for lifting the arch over a period of six weeks[13].

- **Use this towel exercise to strengthen your feet:** There's a great exercise you can use to further fortify your feet and protect your lower limbs from undue stress. The best part is that it is a simple exercise to do while working at your desk or sitting in front of the TV. All you need to make it work is a towel (plus a little bit of brain power to get those muscles activating). Take your shoes and socks off, then place the towel underneath your toes. Now, your task is to scrunch the towel up using your toes until you've pulled in the entire towel. Once you've fully pulled the towel in using just your toes, use your hands to unfurl it again and repeat three times. Don't be surprised if you get a seriously achy pair of feet following this exercise!

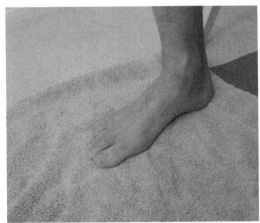

Start sitting in a chair, barefoot, with one foot on the edge of a towel that is laid out on the floor.

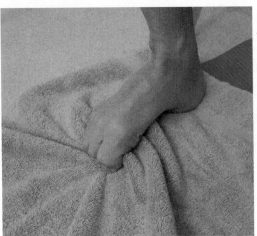

Keeping your heel on the floor at all times, use the muscles in your foot and toes to scrunch the towel up and draw it in towards you. Keep repeating until the towel is fully collected up by your foot, then unravel and repeat 2-3 times on each foot.

The Back Pain Golden Rule

In my years of experience working as a physiotherapist, there's one principle I apply to my back pain treatment programmes that I feel has added more value to my patient's lives than possibly any other. The best part about it is that it's unbelievably simple, yet hardly ever considered by the majority of my patients or their previous healthcare providers. I call it the Back Pain Golden Rule.

If you're currently suffering with back pain, you've probably noticed that some movements or positions are especially painful. For many people, bending forward to pick something up from the floor is the most painful action they can do. For others, leaning back brings them the most discomfort. However, you'll probably also find that some movements of your spine don't cause you as much pain, and may even provide you some temporary relief.

My Golden Rule is simply to only give my clients exercises that involve the *comfortable* movements of their spine, while *avoiding* any aggravating movements until things start to improve.

In this way, I can help my clients to restore the mobility of their spines, reduce stiffness and control their pain while minimising the risk of making symptoms worse. Anyone who has suffered for any length of time knows that it's quite easy to find an exercise that has the opposite to the desired effect and makes their pain worse rather than better, while it can be quite challenging to find an exercise that doesn't hurt and helps them to feel better. My Golden Rule improves the chances that you'll choose an exercise that is helpful rather than harmful.

So, how can you put the Golden Rule into action?

The first step is to work out exactly which movements make your pain worse and which movements improve (or at least don't worsen) your symptoms. Once you've chosen the movements or actions that make your pain better, just try to build them into your daily routine several times per day. I usually tell my clients to choose a nice, comfortable movement and repeat it between 3 and 10 times in a row, every 2-3 hours. This formula tends to work quite well. However, be sure to get your chosen exercise checked by a healthcare professional before you get started, just to check it's appropriate and safe for your problem first.

Once my clients' symptoms start to improve over a number of weeks, I will very slowly try to re-introduce some of the initially painful movements to their routine, in order to re-expose them to those once-problematic movement patterns and protect them from future harm. In a nutshell, along with a good deal of hands-on therapy if appropriate, that is my approach to treating my clients with back pain!

CHAPTER FIVE

Hips & Knees

Introduction

If backs are the most common body part that I treat, knees come in as a close second. The reason I combine hips and knees together in this chapter is because of their close affinity to one another. They have a very strong relationship. For many people who seek me out for help with their knee pain, the root cause of their problem is actually closer to their hips. This also works the other way around. Knowing how closely related these two areas of the body are is the first step to understanding the root cause of a painful problem in either body part.

In this chapter, we're going to dispel some myths about clicking in the hips and knees, how to improve your walking, and my single best exercise for hip and knee strength and health over fifty.

How Your Hips Can Cause Knee Pain

You might be surprised to find that I've put hips and knees together in this section of the book. I can assure you that there's a very good reason for that.

I've already mentioned how our hips and knees are very closely related. They are so closely related, in fact, that when there's a problem with one of these body parts, the other often suffers as well.

I spent a lot of time working with hip and knee injuries when I was working in professional football. I would see lots of knee ligament injuries, groin strains and hamstring problems. One thing that I learned as I continued to work and study was that when one of our players suffered a knee injury, there was often a problem (weakness, tightness or stiffness) in the hip above that knee that preceded the injury.

Sometimes, there was even a problem in the opposite hip instead.

I see the same thing in my clinic now, too, even in people who have never stepped foot onto a football pitch. I see people who come in to see me with a hip problem, but when I look at the knee below, it's also stiff and sore. This means that I often end up helping people with an entirely different problem than the one they thought they'd come in with!

I think it's important for me to explain to you how a hip problem can affect your knees, because this is something that took me a while to get my head around.

When I use the term "hip problem", I mean weakness, stiffness or tightness around the hip joint. It's entirely possible that you wouldn't even know that you've got a problem like this in your hip, because weakness, stiffness and tightness on their own don't always cause pain. However, after a number of months, these issues can lead to imbalances in the muscles around the hip joint. Imbalances can cause the long bone in your thigh (the femur) to fail to "align" properly when you walk, run or climb stairs. And it is *this* problem that can lead to knee pain.

As the upper half of the knee joint is made up of the bottom end of the femur, if the muscles at the hip that control that bone aren't doing their job properly, it is going to affect the alignment of both the hip and the knee. That is why a problem in the hip can cause knee pain.

We can also think about it in the opposite way; if there's a problem around the knee joint (bottom part of the thigh bone), this is going to affect the top part of the thigh bone and may lead to hip pain.

We sometimes even see pain in the right knee due to a problem in the left hip, just to make matters even more confusing! Because the hips make up part of your pelvis, if one side isn't doing its job properly the whole pelvis can drop subtly to one side. This can put an unusual pressure on both legs and may even lead to pain in the opposite side.

So, what can we do to address this problem?

The first step is to diagnose the root cause of the problem and check whether it's a true knee injury or whether an imbalance in the hips is the cause of the problem instead. For that, it's important to be checked out by someone who knows what they're looking for. I'd always recommend getting checked out by a physiotherapist for this, but there are also some clues you can look for at home to tell if your hip is at fault for your knee pain. For example, if you look at the way you move as you sit down and stand up from a chair, does one of your knees fall inwards slightly? Ask a friend or partner to watch and check for you. If they notice one knee slightly rolling inwards, that can be a sign of weakness in your hip.

Once the problem has been identified, a targeted exercise programme with or without some hands-on treatment can be the best remedy. This often means that the majority of your treatment may be focussed on your hips, even though your complaint is knee pain. Don't worry - once the hip imbalance improves, the knee should also get better!

Most of my clients who come to see me for this problem are relieved to hear that it isn't arthritis or a cartilage problem causing their knee pain. In fact, for many people with this type of knee pain, if we X-rayed or scanned their knee, we wouldn't be able to see a problem at all. There doesn't always need to be physical damage for us to feel pain[1]. The type of pain felt in this problem is caused by physical stress over a sustained period of time. You can't "*see*" this kind of injury but you can definitely feel it.

The key is being aware of this common phenomenon and acting early to ensure it doesn't develop into a bigger problem. Acting early can help to prevent problems later down the line, and nip any painful stresses and strains in the bud before they get worse.

Now, we're going to talk about another extremely common yet poorly understood problem: clicking knees.

The Truth About Clicking Knees

By far, one of the most common things I get asked is *"Why do my knees click all the time?"*

This question is usually asked by a concerned patient who has some knee pain that they are managing quite well - but the constant orchestra coming from their knees is making them doubt their progress. Clicking, clunking and grinding inside your knee can truly be an alarming symptom! The unpleasant natural image that it conjures up is that of bone grinding against bone every time you move your knee joint.

However, one thing I can assure you is that this is rarely the cause of clicking knees.

First, let's quickly recap how the joints in our body work so we can understand what causes clicking in the knees. Our joints are made up of the meeting place between two or more bones. Between these bones is a wonderful substance called cartilage. Cartilage acts as a shock absorber and a lubricant, making sure the two bones don't come into close contact with each other. Another substance, a fluid called synovial fluid, works with the cartilage to provide lubrication between the bones and allow the joint to move freely.

Over time, we sometimes find that the cartilage in our joints can become uneven and form tiny channels on its surface. Clicking can often occur as the synovial fluid rushes through these tiny channels, with the air bubbles within the fluid popping to give you that clicking sounds that can be so disturbing. If you've ever felt like you've got "sand" inside your knee joint, this is also the most likely culprit behind that sensation.

Another cause of clicking knees for some people is the fact that their knee cap isn't moving as it was designed to. When the knee cap is functioning perfectly, it slides directly up and down in the groove that nature created on our thigh bone. However, if we are weak in some key muscles and tight in others, the knee cap doesn't slide perfectly up and down any more because of the uneven pull caused by these muscles[2]. What we often see is a knee cap "tracking" off to one side, and because the knee cap has left its groove, the movement isn't perfect any longer and clicking can be heard as a result.

Just as I mentioned in the previous chapter, it isn't always the knee muscles that are at fault. This problem is yet another issue that can be caused by weakness in your hips. If your hip muscles aren't strong enough to keep your thigh bone in line, your knee falls inwards and the knee cap can't move as it was designed to any longer. This can lead to knee cap pain and clicking, even though the real underlying issue is up in the hip[3].

It's very rare for clicking knees to be caused by bone rubbing against bone. Usually, bone rubbing against bone would be so painful that you'd be unable to walk, let alone put enough pressure through your legs to set off the clicking in your knees. This means that I am usually able to put my clients' minds at ease when they come to me worrying that their knee has deteriorated and that they are going to need to be rushed through for urgent surgery.

However, as with all other problems mentioned in this book, it's best to get checked out by a professional if you're worried. Hopefully, your mind will be put at ease too.

Clicking knees don't necessarily mean that you've got arthritis, either. I used to treat young girls as young as 16 years of age coming to my clinic with the noisiest knees you've ever heard. The noise wasn't because their joints are deteriorating. It was simply because their knee cap wasn't quite moving correctly. Luckily, this is a problem that we are very good at fixing for people.

One important caveat to mention is that although clicking doesn't mean your knees are degenerating, if left for an extended period of time there is a possibility that your long-term knee health could suffer[4]. Knee clicking generally means there is an issue with movement at that joint, and when a joint isn't moving properly it leaves the cartilage vulnerable to wear and tear over a long period of time.

You can think of clicking knees as an early warning sign that your movement isn't quite right. The good news is that, more often than not, these problems can be fixed when caught early! The key is early detection and swift action: if you've got noisy knees, get them checked to safeguard against problems in the future.

Do Your Hips Swivel?

One of the hobbies most commonly enjoyed by my clients is golf.

Most people know that you need to be able to twist from your lower back to be able to hit the ball straight and far. But did you also know that being able to rotate at your hips is also crucial for a proper golf swing[5]?

Without being able to rotate your hips, it would be impossible to get a proper follow-through with any golf swing. Your trailing leg wouldn't be able to turn to allow your body to follow the ball as you swing through.

It isn't just your golf game that would be affected without the capacity for proper hip rotation. Swimming, walking and bowls would be very difficult without good hip mobility. At the extreme, without the ability to rotate at your hips, you will start to find even putting your socks on and getting into a car challenging.

I meet some clients who get groin pain when they get up after sitting for a long time in the car or at home. On closer inspection, they've lost a great deal of their capacity for hip rotation, which can cause aches and pains when you start moving again after being at rest. If this sounds like you, it's important to act before your hips get any stiffer.

Most people have some degree of arthritis in their hips by the time they reach their 50th birthday[6]. Arthritis usually leads to a loss of hip rotation, long before the first signs of pain. This means that you could be affected by this loss of hip movement without even knowing it!

However, no need to worry just yet. With a little time and practice, it is possible to regain some of the rotation around your hips and get the swivel back in your step.

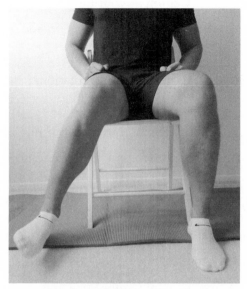

Internal rotation of the hip

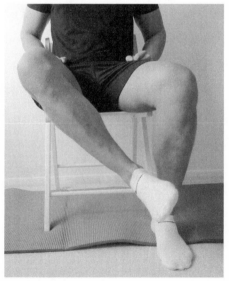

External rotation of the hip

There are two types of rotation at your hip joint. If you sit in a chair and turn your thigh so that you are bringing the inside of your shin up towards you and your foot off the floor (as if you were putting your socks on), you're performing the first type of hip rotation, called external rotation.

If you do the opposite movement, turning your thigh bone so that the outside of your shin comes up towards you while your foot comes off the floor (as if you're trying to touch the outside of your heel), that is the second type of hip rotation, called internal rotation.

We used to believe that there was a pattern of movement deterioration with arthritis. The early researchers believed people would almost always lose internal rotation first. However, more recent research shows this to not necessarily be the case[7].

While you may find that you struggle with at least one of these movements, it is possible to notice at least some improvements in the range of motion at the hip joint simply by practicing these actions from a sitting position, consistently over a long period of time. It does take time and you may progress so slowly that you hardly notice, but most of my clients who stick to working on these movements do realise over time that getting into a car becomes easier, they have less trouble with socks and, sometimes, their golf game even improves too!

The exercise on the following pages can be done very carefully to avoid aggravating already-painful hips, but it's worth speaking to a doctor or physiotherapist before putting this one into action. For hips that are painful, just move within a comfortable range. If you have hips that aren't painful but are very stiff, you could try gently pushing into these stiff ranges and slowly building up. Stop at any point if you develop pain in the hip or groin. If you've been given the all clear by your physiotherapist, try the gentle exercise below to regain some of your hip movement:

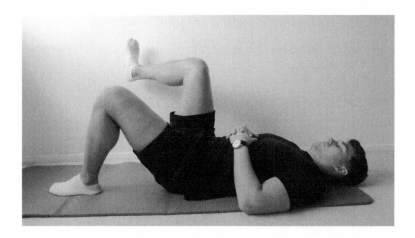

Start lying on your back on the bed or the floor. Bring one knee up so your foot is off the floor. Then, keeping your knee at 90 degrees, rotate your leg first internally (top picture), then externally (bottom picture). Repeat 10 times each direction slowly, for 3 sets.

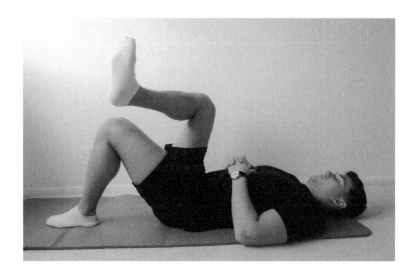

Trouble with Walking? Look to Your Pelvis

For you to be able to walk well, there must be synergy between your feet, ankles, knees and hips. These joints all move in unison to propel us forward as we walk. When we take a step, we begin by generating tension in our foot as it strikes the ground. Strong hip muscles then work to drive our leg behind us as our knee muscles work to extend our knee. Finally, our calf muscles propel us forward as we push off through our toes.

None of this movement would be possible if we didn't have a solid, stable foundation to produce these actions from. This solid, stable foundation is your pelvis.

If we don't have good pelvic control, we can't expect our walking to be as comfortable or efficient as we'd like it to be. The fact is, many people have lost control of their pelvis without knowing it. This can be a common cause of walking problems, hip problems and even back pain[8].

So, how can you tell if you've got a problem with controlling your pelvis? One easy way is to try and move your pelvis and take note of how easy (or difficult) it may be.

To do this, start off standing with your hands on your hips. Without moving your lower back or your knees, can you roll your pelvis forwards, sticking your bottom out? And now can you roll your pelvis backwards, tucking your tailbone between your legs and pulling your bottom in?

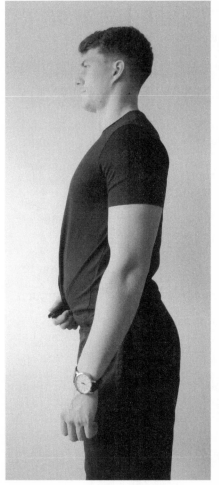
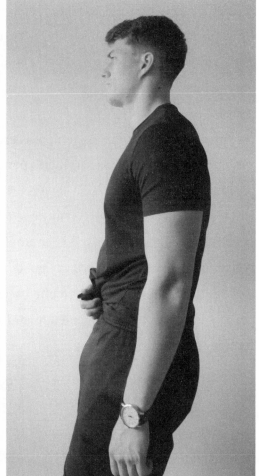

| Anterior pelvic tilt | Posterior pelvic tilt |

If these movements seem foreign or difficult to you, there's a high probability that your pelvic control isn't up to scratch.

Many people can do one of these pelvic movements but not the other. If this is the case, it's likely that your posture has changed and you're favouring one of these tilted pelvic positions when you stand and walk.

There are many ways to correct this, but working on rolling the pelvis forwards and backwards from a variety of positions is a great place to start. You might want to spend a few minutes every day practicing rolling your pelvis forwards and backwards when sitting, standing, and lying on your back.

You will find that the movement is easier or more difficult for you in certain positions. Continue trying to perform the action in the difficult positions as this is where you'll gain the most benefit.

Once you feel that you've "loosened up" your stiff pelvis, you may notice that your back, hip and knee troubles are a lot easier. You may notice that you can walk further than before. You may notice that you tire less easily. All of these positive effects can come from just a few minutes per day of practicing a movement that, for most people, has become foreign to them.

Knee Cap Pain - What's Behind It?

Pain at the front of the knee is an incredibly common problem for many people, young and old. I'd go as far as saying that in the young people I see in my clinic, it is possibly the most common problem I help them with.

However, knee cap pain doesn't just affect young people. This problem equally affects over-fifties too. Even though arthritis can sometimes be involved with knee cap pain in over-fifties's, the same problem that causes the pain in a sixteen-year-old can be the culprit in a sixty-year-old too.

Knee cap pain usually occurs due to a problem with the way that your knee cap is moving[9]. Your knee cap was built to sit in a "groove" on top of the long leg bone in your thigh (called your femur). As you bend and straighten your knee, your knee cap slides up and down on top of this bone - acting like a pulley system - allowing your knee muscles to pull on your shin bone and create movement.

Your knee cap has certain muscles that attach onto it and pull it in different directions. When everything is balanced, the knee cap is pulled directly up and down inside the groove and you have healthy knee movement. However, when some of these muscles pull either too hard or not hard enough, the knee cap may start to slide up and down outside of the centre of the groove. When this happens, knee cap pain can be the result.

There is a little pocket of fat called a "fat pad" that sits underneath the knee cap. This fat pad acts as a cushion and lubricates movement. It also has nerves within it, so when the fat pad gets irritated (by the knee cap not moving correctly), it can become very inflamed and painful.

Knee cap pain is often felt *behind* the knee cap and it can feel as if you want to get in behind the knee cap and add some WD40 at times! While adding WD40 to your joints isn't practical unfortunately, there are some things you can do to relieve knee pain with this problem. We'll go over some of my best tips for doing just that in a moment.

One of the most important things to do first, however, is to get assessed by a movement specialist like a physiotherapist. They can assess which muscles are pulling too hard and which aren't pulling enough, then show you what to do to fix it.

In some cases, knee cap pain is due to arthritis, but try not to worry just yet! Arthritis symptoms can often be greatly improved through conservative measures, without needing to opt for surgery, injections or pain killers.

Here are some top tips for easing knee cap pain at home:

• **Try using ice over the knee cap when it's painful:** You can apply a cold compress or ice pack to a painful knee cap to relieve some of the pain. Ice is nature's painkiller and it is very effective for knee cap pain as the problem tends to sit close to the surface. This approach can help to calm an irritated fat pad underneath the knee cap. Be sure to protect the skin and treat your knee with ice for no longer than 15-minutes at a time.

- **Try using heat on the muscles around the knee:** The muscles above the knee at the front of your thigh can become sore, stiff and painful when you've got knee cap pain. Using a hot water bottle or warm compress on these areas can provide some relief. Again, protect the skin and treat for 15-minutes at a time.

- **Try to move in a straight line:** When we get up from a sitting position, often we're in a rush to do something, so we turn as we're rising from the chair. Try not to do this if you've got knee cap pain. When you twist while getting up from a chair, you can accidentally aggravate your knee cap by causing it to move outside of its groove.

- **If walking is painful, try walking in the swimming pool for exercise:** When we're walking on land, we take 100% of our body weight through our legs. In the absence of a painful problem, this is fine. However, when you're suffering with knee pain, your body weight suddenly feels much heavier! If taking your weight through your knees is giving you discomfort but you still want to get some all-important exercise in, try walking for 30-minutes in the swimming pool instead. When submerged in the water, 50% of your body weight is offloaded onto the water so you only need to carry the other 50% through your joints. This should result in instant relief compared to walking on land. The good thing about walking in the water is that it's fantastic exercise as you're constantly pushing forward against water resistance. This means you're able to build strength (very important) without worsening your pain in doing so.

• **Try to lose some weight:** If you're a little on the heavy side at the moment, losing weight should significantly improve your symptoms[10]. I understand it can be very difficult to lose weight when you're in pain because of how hard this makes it to exercise. However, just a small change in your body weight can be noticed as a dramatic improvement in symptoms. As a general rough rule, I usually start to see noticeable improvements in my clients' knee pain symptoms following around 2kg (4.4lbs) of weight loss. You can find more information about losing weight with a painful problem later in the book on page 236.

"No Hands!" The Key to Maintaining Knee Strength Past Fifty

There is one thing that scares people of my grandparent's generation like nothing else. It strips people of their independence and can land them in the hospital, sometimes for days on end. Some unfortunately never make it back out. Any idea what I'm referring to? I'm talking about falls.

A fall can be absolutely catastrophic; not just for the elderly, but for anyone of middle age and beyond. All it takes is one unfortunate landing and you could suffer a fractured hip, broken wrist or dislocated shoulder. Any of these injuries can cause significant disability and pain, for a very long time in some cases. During my time working in the NHS, I saw hundreds of patients following a fall that had led to a significant injury, many still struggling months later. Most of these people did eventually recover, but many had life-long disability resulting from that one fall.

I've also seen the aftermath of falls in my own family - with my Grandmother suffering severe bruises all over after falling at home.

For me, that alone has been motivation enough to try and help whoever I can to avoid these terrifying falls. People fall for many reasons and sometimes falls are unavoidable. However, two of the most common reasons for falling in people over fifty are **poor balance** and a **loss of strength in the legs**.[11]

As we grow older, we do tend to lose some of our ability to balance. It would be unusual for someone to be able to stand on one leg at seventy as well as they could when they were thirty. However, this is mostly due to the effect of de-training. When we get older and face the inevitable "slowing down" that comes with later life, our balance is no longer challenged to the extent that it used to be. The human body has a very predictable way of becoming inefficient at the things that we don't practice regularly. If we don't practice balancing outside of our comfort zones from time to time, we'll have no balancing ability to draw on to correct us if we stumble across a challenge in our day-to-day lives.

In these situations, with someone whose lost their ability to balance, it often only takes the slightest trip to cause a fall. However, if they had been regularly practice balancing at home, they'd be able to correct themselves without much bother, avoiding that fall all together.

On the flip side, sometimes I'll get a patient over fifty who comes into my office for their painful problem and when I test their balance, they have phenomenal ability to stand on one leg. More often than not, when I marvel at how good they are (sometimes able to stand on one leg with their eyes closed) they smile wryly and tell me about the Yoga class they've attend every week for the past decade. These people rarely fall, even in older age. This proves that with regular practice, you can significantly improve your balance, even beyond sixty years of age.

While heading to the directory to find your nearest Yoga class would be a good idea for many reading this, it isn't necessary to get the benefits I'm describing. There are some effective methods that can be put into action at home to improve your balance, starting today:

• **Practice your balance at home:** When practicing balance tasks at home, you should always ensure your safety by starting off holding onto the kitchen work top or the back of a chair until you find your feet. Never practice balance out of the reach of something that you can quickly grab hold of to steady yourself if necessary. Always start slow and build up - it should initially feel a little challenging but not impossible. Some good options for practicing your balance include standing with your feet very close together and taking your fingers away from the worktop, one by one. If you can do this for 30-seconds with no bother, progress to standing with your feet in line, right heel touching left toes (as if walking a tightrope), then repeat the above. If you can do this for 30-seconds, you can practice standing on one leg. I usually tell people to start holding onto the worktop with both hands, then take away their hand support, finger by finger. Once you feel steady and you've only got one finger on the worktop, try taking your hand off altogether. When you practice balancing in this way, be sure to always have someone nearby who can watch you and make sure that you're safe. As with any exercise in this book, be sure to be checked over by a doctor or physiotherapist for suitability before giving it a try.

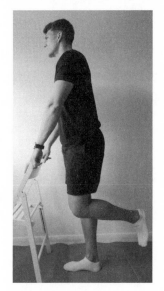

• **Practice getting up and out of a chair:** While your balancing ability is very important in avoiding falls, having significant strength in your lower limbs is crucial as well[11]. One of the simplest, yet most effective ways of building and maintaining leg strength is by practicing sitting down and standing up from a chair. By completing the movement without using your hands and being sure to sit down as slowly as you possibly can (taking around 4-seconds to go from standing to sitting is good), you're going to build significant strength in your hips and knees, safeguarding you from falls as a result of your knees or hips giving way. Do not proceed with any exercise (including this one) if it is painful, and be sure to start from a higher chair (which should be easier) before trying this exercise from low chairs.

Working on your balance takes time; don't expect to see a huge improvement in the first few weeks. As with anything worth having, progress takes effort and plenty of days of consistent practice. However, I've yet to meet someone who tells me that avoiding a fractured hip and maintaining their independence in later life isn't worth a little hard work!

The Truth About Knee Arthritis

If you're over fifty, chances are that you can't get ten minutes into a conversation with a group of close friends before someone brings up an ache, pain or even surgery that they've had because of arthritis.

There's a lot of doom and gloom in the media about arthritis too. The press also often use poorly designed research studies to sell papers with headlines that read something like *"The Newest Arthritis Wonder Cure!"*… Only for us to read several lines in that the dubious study being quoted found that there was a slight, tenuous link between some household item and minor pain relief from arthritis, in a specific, niche subset of people.

But what *really* does it mean to have arthritis? Is it a life sentence of pain, misery and suffering?

I would argue that it is not.

Arthritis, in medical terms, is the deterioration of the cartilage in a joint due to the process of ageing. However, how this is *experienced* differs dramatically from person to person.

You might assume that when your cartilage starts to deteriorate, you automatically become stiff and your joints get extremely painful. This is not necessarily true. In recent studies where people over fifty have been put through an MRI scanner, the results show that almost everyone suffers from some degree of arthritis[12]. Somewhat surprisingly, only a fraction of these people report any pain.

I have had too many clients to count who have come to see me for an entirely separate painful problem, only to have a scan done that picked up an incidental finding of severe arthritis in another area of the body; an area that has never given them any trouble whatsoever.

How can this be? How can some people suffer so badly, while others seem to get away with it, Scott free?

The short answer is, we don't fully understand the answer to this question yet. There are certainly some factors that can make pain in arthritis more likely. For example, if you are overweight and there's more pressure traveling through an arthritic joint, it would make sense that this would lead to pain in some cases[13].

One other thing that has become clear to me during my years of practice is that if you take two people, one with stiff joints and the other with no stiffness, the one with the stiffness tends to suffer with worse pain than the one who has better movement, even if the degree of arthritis in that joint is the same in those two people[14]. This is certainly the case when we talk about knees. When someone comes to me for treatment of their knee arthritis, the first thing I look at is whether they can fully bend and straighten their knee. If they can't, that's the first thing I look to restore for them, and more often than not, that improves their symptoms reasonably quickly.

One thing that I look to help people avoid in my work as a physiotherapist is the need to go under the knife for a total knee replacement. Most of my clients value living without the fear of risky surgery and I work towards helping them achieve that goal. While there's no denying that the work orthopaedic surgeons do with people's knees these days is nothing short of incredible, at the time of writing, even the best total knee replacement will only last 10-15 years at a maximum before it needs "revising". These revisions are never as straightforward as the first time around, so delaying surgery for as long as possible the first time around is very important.

Even after your first total knee replacement surgery, the recovery process can be long and painful. It's a significant, major surgery; it should never be taken lightly. Total knee replacement surgery can be risky and I always maintain that it should be a last resort.

If you can feel the rumblings of knee arthritis, which usually feels like a dull ache around the sides of your knee joint, there are some things you can do to ease the pain and improve your mobility without having to reach for the pain killers or rush to see your orthopaedic surgeon:

- **Try to maintain a full range of movement at your knee joint:** If you struggle to press the back of your knee down into the bed when you're lying on your back, or you're unable to fully bend your knee so your heel touches your bottom, you've currently got a stiff knee joint. Stiff knees are often painful, but when this problem is corrected, symptoms usually improve to a degree regardless of the underlying arthritis still remaining. You could practice gently bending and straightening your knee for several minutes each day to build some flexibility back into the knee joint. Over a number of weeks, you should notice a difference on stairs and getting into and out of chairs.

- **Use a warm compress on the knee in the morning:** If you suffer like many others with morning stiffness in your knee for the first 15-minutes or so upon getting out of bed, the first thing you should do as part of your morning routine is make a hot water bottle. By warming up the knee joint with a hot water bottle or hot bath, you can start to relieve stiffness and pain far quicker than if you wait for the area to "heat up" naturally. You can also use this method whenever you're suffering from stiffness and pain, as is more often the case in the winter months.

• **Keep active, keep walking:** When in pain, staying active can be difficult, especially when the alternative is sitting by the fire with your feet up. However, continuing to walk regularly is especially important for those with arthritis. One reason for this is that having weak knee muscles contributes to the pain when there's some wear to the cartilage in your knees. Researchers from the University of Korea, Seoul, found that those with less leg muscle experienced worse pain with knee arthritis[15]. By walking regularly, you can minimise the rate of muscle loss in your legs and keep those knee joints well-protected. The old adage *"if you don't use it, you lose it"* is very true when it comes to walking. It won't be long before disuse leads to lack of ability to go on those long hikes, sometimes permanently if you're not careful. Keep active, keep walking, keep those legs as strong as you can.

• **Ask your doctor about capsaicin cream:** Capsaicin cream is a reasonably new product in Western medicine, but its arthritis relieving qualities have been known about in the Far East for many centuries. Capsaicin is one of the substances in chilli peppers that gives them their heat, and applying this substance in the form of a cream to the skin over an arthritic joint has been shown to provide effective relief for many people[16]. Capsaicin cream is unfortunately a prescription-only medicine in the UK at the time of writing, but if you ask your GP for some they are usually happy to oblige.

The Truth About Hip Arthritis

The fact that arthritis can occur in the absence of pain is as true when it comes to your hips as it is with your knees. However, pain from hip arthritis can be truly debilitating for some people, affecting their quality of life even more so, arguably, than knee arthritis.

Hip arthritis usually shows up as pain in the groin rather than on the outside of the hip, although the latter can occasionally occur. You might feel a restriction in your hip joint, or notice more clicking and clunking than usual. Walking in hilly areas may become more challenging. In the later stages of hip arthritis, some people report a scary sensation of "giving way" at the hip, as if their muscles suddenly refuse to support them any longer.

In terms of treatment, the same principles apply for hip arthritis as for knee arthritis; remaining strong in the surrounding muscles and keeping your movement capability is key, which is echoed in a recent Cochrane review on the topic of hip arthritis[17]. From my experience, I have seen the general trend that hips can be protected from many of the nasty symptoms of arthritis by maintaining a good range of motion.

What does a good range of motion in the hips look like? Well, for a start, you should be able to put your socks on and off without too much trouble. You should also be able to get in and out of a low car seat without feeling stiffness or tightness in your hip or groin.

If you struggle with either of these daily tasks, it's a good idea to arrange to see someone who can help you with improving the movement in your hips as quickly as you possibly can, to prevent the problem from progressing any further. This may come as a surprise, but even if you've started to lose mobility in your hips, it isn't necessarily the start of a downward spiral into declining mobility - provided that you do something about it early. Through certain hands-on methods, some physiotherapists have developed ways to improve hip mobility and maintain good hip health, despite the effects of ageing, while exercises also help.

The other incredibly useful approach we can take with people suffering from this condition is to help them strengthen the muscles that support the hip joint. This can "offload" the joint and help to stop that horrible "giving way" sensation.

One big difference that exists between hip and knee arthritis is what you can expect following joint replacement surgery with the two conditions. Knee replacement surgery is more complex and carries a longer recovery time (as well as possibly more pain and disability in the first six weeks after the operation), while hip replacement surgery is usually simpler with a smoother recovery. Either way, both are major surgeries and should be regarded as such.

At my clinic, we have many health-conscious clients who are admirably determined to take their health into their own hands, refusing to rely on medical procedures as a means for "fixing" age-related aches and pains. The results we are able to get with some of these clients is amazing and shows the potential for improvement in hip arthritis without always necessarily needing to undergo risky surgery.

The Single Best Hip & Knee Exercise

While most of my clients value their health greatly, they also value anything that is going to save them time and unnecessary energy. By the time you reach the age of fifty, you've probably come to the realisation that your time is far too valuable to waste on things that aren't adding value to your life.

That's why, when it comes to health and my approach with my clients, I always prioritise the strategies, tips and exercises that are going to give my clients the biggest "bang for their buck", from a time perspective. Less is often more. So, for this chapter, I thought I'd show you the single most valuable exercise you can possibly do for your hips and knees, to maintain strength and function throughout the rest of your life.

After a lot of careful thought, I can confidently say that if I had to give you one exercise to do daily for the remainder of your days in order to improve your quality of life as much as I possibly could, this exercise would be it.

We call this exercise the *"Goblet Squat"* and I've chosen it for its practicality, ease of use and the incredible benefits it provides. The Goblet Squat falls into the category of a "compound exercise": one that uses multiple joints and muscles. We perform some variation of the Goblet Squat most days without even realising it. Simply getting up and out of a chair without using your hands is the starting variation of the Goblet Squat, and is the place I recommend most people start.

As with all the exercises in this book, this exercise won't be suitable for everyone; you should be sure to be checked over by your doctor or physiotherapist before adding this to any daily routine.

In the pictures below, you'll see a demonstration of the Goblet Squat.

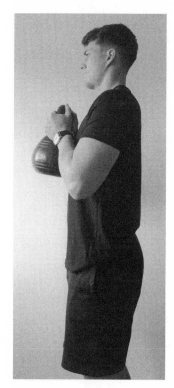
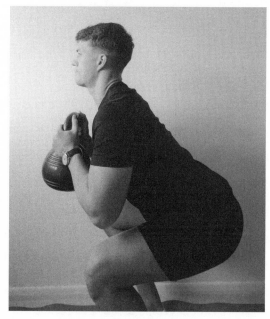

Start standing, holding a weight or a bag of books close to your chest. Keeping your back straight, bend at the hips and knees as if to sit back. Slowly sink down as low as you can comfortably (never into pain) then stand back up again. Complete 10-15 repetitions of this exercise, rest for a minute, then repeat 2 or 3 times. If you can do more than 15 repetitions with ease, find something a little heavier to hold.

To perform this exercise correctly, you need to hinge at both the hips and the knees. The two muscle groups responsible for controlling this hinging action are the muscles in the buttock area (called the "gluteals") and the muscles at the front of the thigh (called the "quadriceps"). These are the main muscles that work to allow us to walk and stand without our knees or hips giving way - thus, by strengthening them further, we improve every activity that involves standing or being on our feet (i.e. almost everything!)

You'll also see in the picture that we use a small weight held in front of us near to our chest. This is what gives the exercise the name "Goblet Squat", because it involves holding a dumbbell as if it were a goblet in front of the body (it's an old fashioned term, granted). By holding a dumbbell, you're adding some extra resistance which challenges the hip and knee muscles further and builds strength more than just performing the exercise with your bodyweight. However, you may need to start with just your bodyweight in order to get going, then progress from there.

To make this exercise easier or harder, you can choose whether or not your bottom makes contact with a seat when you drop down to the lowest point. If you were to make contact with the seat, it would take the tension off the muscles for a while and should make the exercise easier, in theory. However, in practice, this will take away all momentum from your movement during the exercise and may actually make it feel harder (as you'll be standing up again from the chair from a completely still-start). Either way, the exercise works fabulously for improving your mobility and strength and translates well to many activities that we perform every day without thinking; such as walking, getting in and out of a car, climbing stairs and picking things up from the floor.

I always recommend working in a pain-free range and building up from there, trying to increase the depth of the squat as time goes on and movement becomes more comfortable.

Start by performing a set of 5-10 repetitions and then building up to 15 repetitions in a row. If you can do 15 with no problem, find something slightly heavier to hold in front of you (you do not necessarily need to go and invest in a set of dumbbells; a big book would be a good starting point).

Pain on the Side of Your Hip? Here's the Plan...

In my clinic at HT Physio, I very regularly see people (especially women over fifty) come in suffering from pain at the side of their hip, that just doesn't seem to get any better no matter what they try.

A lot of people assume that this must be the first signs of hip arthritis rearing its ugly head. However, more often than not, this pain is caused by something entirely different.

It's true that pain on the side of your hip can sometimes be "referred"; caused by a problem in your lower back. However, there is an entirely different problem that is more often the culprit.

Most cases of pain at the side of the hip are caused by an injury to the tendons around the side of the hip, or inflammation of a little fluid sac around this area (known as "bursitis"). We used to try and tell these two problems apart, but we don't any longer. Instead, we give them a very fancy collective name, called *"greater trochanteric pain syndrome"* (or GTPS).

GTPS is just a clever term for pain around the bony area on the side of your hip (called the greater trochanter). It is characterised by:

- Tenderness to touch around the side of your hip
- Pain when walking and standing
- Difficulty standing on one leg
- Pain on stairs
- Pain walking up or down hills

GTPS is a very common problem - in fact, research shows us that it will affect 10-25% of the population[18], making it as common as hip arthritis - and it can be just as debilitating in many cases. We see it a lot more commonly in women than in men. This is because a difference in the shape of our pelvises. Women tend to have wider set pelvises (think of the traditional "hourglass" shape of a woman's curves) than men, and this puts the tendons in the hip onto a stretch which can predispose the fairer sex to GTPS. Sorry, ladies!

A very subtle, long-standing weakness that affects the way you walk or stand can lead to repetitive strain on these tendons and on the area over the side of your hip. This repetitive strain leads to tiny tears in the tendons and inflammation in the little fluid sac (called a bursa) on the side of your hip, which can lead to GTPS.

In most cases of this problem, weakness of the hip muscles precedes the start of pain[19]. Women require more hip muscle strength than men to walk properly (again, because of the differences in the way their pelvises are built) but most of the ladies I assess in clinic, candidly, have poor hip muscle strength. This leaves them at risk of problems like GTPS.

However, if you've developed pain on the side of your hip, it isn't too late to address the deficits in your hip strength. In fact, restoring the strength of the hip muscles is actually one of the best ways to treat GTPS. I'm afraid that, as everyone with this problem has hip weakness that behaves in slightly different ways, it would be difficult for me to show you exactly what to do to strengthen the hips in this book (as it's very easy to make your pain worse by doing even slightly the wrong thing). However, the next pages should still be of some help. There are some absolutely must-know "rules" when it comes to this condition that, when obeyed, can dramatically improve your rate of recovery:

- With GTPS, getting comfortable at night can be a challenge. If you're going to lie on your side at night, **consider lying on top of a soft duvet** which can 'cushion' the area below your hip and prevent pressure from aggravating the injury.

- If you're going to lie on your opposite side at night, be sure to **place a pillow between your legs**. This is important. Letting your legs cross over the midline of your body compresses the painful area (even when you don't directly feel pain from it) and can prevent the problem from getting better. Most of us are side sleepers, so we run the risk of spending eight hours every night with our bad leg crossed over mid-line - not good for our hips! By placing a pillow between your legs, you can ensure the bad leg doesn't cross over the mid-line of the body which should relieve some pressure from the painful area.

- **Don't "hip hang"!** Most of us are guilty of this; shifting from one foot to the other while standing, chatting away to a friend. The problem with this is that as we place all of our weight on one leg, our hips move over to one side, increasing pressure on the affected area as we "hang" by our hips. Again, this can aggravate GTPS, so make sure you stand with your weight spread evenly between your feet, at least until the painful problem settles down.

- This might be the hardest habit to break, but it's incredibly important: **You need to stop crossing your legs!** When you cross your legs when sitting or even lying on your back, you put pressure through the painful area which aggravates the side of your hip. This is one of the biggest causes of the problem in the first place, and chronic leg-crossing definitely prevents a lot of people from getting better as fast as they should. Be sure to avoid crossing your legs - if necessary, ask a partner to remind you to uncross every time they see you do so.

- **Try to avoid very low chairs** - by sitting in low chairs, you're asking your hip muscles to work very hard to lift you back out of the chair. The pressure from this action can aggravate the problem and cause a lot of pain. Try placing a pillow under your bottom when sitting in the low chairs around your house to save yourself.

- **Try to avoid standing on one leg** - you may laugh at this one but a lot of us do exactly that every day when we put on and take off our trousers, shoes and socks! Make sure you get dressed while sitting whenever possible if you don't do so already.

- **Avoid extra long walks or going up and down hills where possible.** You may find that walking aggravates your hip pain and you struggle to walk as far as you once could. When suffering from

GTPS, "*no pain, no gain*" is not a sensible approach. You should listen to what your hip is telling you; if it's painful, don't try and push through! Take a break and get back to your walk when it's settled again. Hills are probably the biggest challenge for people with this problem, so try and avoid steep hills where you can. Do try to keep active; however, you may benefit from temporarily cutting down your overall walking distance until the pain settles.

• **Use the handrail whenever climbing stairs.** Stairs are another common daily activity that aggravates GTPS. Try to walk up stairs using the handrail to take a bit of pressure off your hip.

There are certain targeted exercises that are extremely effective at improving the pain associated with GTPS. However, the technique has to be absolutely spot-on for these exercises to be effective, so they are beyond the scope of this book. Be sure to get in touch with a physio early if you're suffering from GTPS so you can get started with a proper rehabilitation programme and recover from this problem as soon as possible.

What to Do When Knee Pain Affects Your Walking

Although I hope that your walking isn't affected by knee pain, realistically there are probably many people reading this section who have knee problems that do stop them from walking as far as they'd like. When knee pain limits walking, it can be debilitating; not just on a physical level but on a social level as well. Walking is a hobby that is commonly enjoyed with friends and loved ones. When this is threatened, those socialising opportunities are threatened as well.

This section of the book is designed to give you information and advice regarding my recommended steps for you to take if you find yourself in a position where your walks aren't as comfortable, or you aren't able to get as far as you'd like.

My first piece of advice to the people I talk to with this problem is to tell them to get checked out so they know exactly what's causing their knee pain. However, as I have mentioned several times in this book, that doesn't necessarily mean that getting an X-ray or MRI scan is the best option. The causes of most knee pain can be diagnosed clinically, either by a physiotherapist or a doctor with experience in assessing knees. There are very subtle differences in signs and symptoms between the causes of knee pain that can easily be missed, so it's important to get assessed by a specialist.

Once you know what's going on, you can formulate a treatment plan designed around your goals and aspirations. If your goal is to be able to walk 20 miles each week, your treatment programme should look decidedly different to someone else whose goals are simply to climb their stairs without pain. If you feel you've been given a generic treatment plan, something isn't right and you should seek a better, more thorough alternative.

Your goals will also dictate the time it takes to achieve an acceptable outcome. If you want to achieve some degree of pain relief, that can usually be done with a few treatments, over the course of several weeks. However, in order to fix the underlying problem and ensure that your knees stay healthy for years to come, a more lengthy time investment is needed as well as more thorough treatment. Either way, your healthcare professional should be able to accommodate your needs and set out a pre-agreed treatment programme with guidance on what to expect at each point throughout the course of your care.

Other than getting one-on-one treatment, if knee pain is affecting your walking, there are a few things that you can do that improve things for almost everyone with this particular problem:

• **Experiment with a knee brace:** While knee supports don't "fix" the underlying problem, they might just help you get through that long walk without being forced to stop. There is conflicting evidence about whether or not they help to prevent twists and sprains[20], but I figure they can't do harm so may be worth considering.

• **If you're into long hikes, try a walking pole:** Almost all of my clients hate the idea of using a walking stick (and the desire to walk independently without needing to use a stick any longer is a common reason my clients approach me in the first place) but using a walking *pole* affords you the support of a stick without the stigma attached to using a true "walking aid". Walking poles are regularly used by all members of the walking community, regardless of age or knee health, and anecdotally reduce knee discomfort on long walks (despite the research showing little to no effect on actual walking mechanics[21]), as well as possibly improving your endurance too. They can be picked up relatively inexpensively from a variety of general or sporting stores and are growing in popularity as each year passes.

- **Keep your knees warm, especially in winter:** If you ever feel like you start off stiff for the first 15 minutes of a walk but then "loosen up" as the walk goes on, you'll probably benefit from *pre-warming* your knees before any kind of walk, as well as keeping your knees warm as you continue. This may involve really blasting the car heater before you start your walk, as well as wearing long-johns or leggings for your walk in the winter. Many of my clients are truly surprised at the difference this tip makes. Letting a sore joint become cold is a sure-fire route to discomfort, so try to avoid it where possible.

- **Substitute a walk for a long cycle ride:** Most of my clients with knee pain while walking actually find cycling pain-free. Cycling is as good, if not better, for building and maintaining cardiovascular fitness and good heart health. You'll also find that it places significantly less stress on your knees than walking or jogging. Dig the bike out of the garage this weekend and give it a try!

• **Build some strength in the swimming pool:** The true conundrum faced by many people with knee pain is that they need to get their legs strong to improve their symptoms - but their knee pain stops them from exercising effectively to do so! As a solution to this problem, I often recommend my clients start a strengthening routine in the swimming pool. The water immediately takes 50% of your body weight away from your lower limbs which is usually enough to diminish any pain felt when walking on land. Walking in the water and swimming lengths is usually a pain-free way of improving your strength (both on land and in the water) that can work wonders for people with knee pain. Start off by walking a few lengths in the water, striding out against the resistance of the water in the pool. You'll find yourself getting tired quicker than you would walking on land (which is a good thing - it means you're challenging yourself). One more thing - be careful with breast stroke. For many people with knee pain, swimming breast stroke can aggravate the problem. Stick to breast-stroke-arms and front-crawl-legs instead.

CHAPTER SIX

Feet & Ankles

Introduction

Your feet aren't just the parts of your body furthest away from you that you lost the ability to reach down and touch several years ago. They are far more important than that. They connect you to the ground and allow you to stand, walk and run with, hopefully, minimal difficulty.

But things can go wrong with our feet and ankles. When things do go wrong in these key areas, it often doesn't take long before we start to suffer in other parts of our body too. Foot problems can lead to ankle problems, which lead to knee problems which can, in turn, cause problems with the back and the hips. Did you think that the toe pain you're currently suffering with is only affecting that one tiny part of your body? Think again.

The facts above about why our feet and ankles are so important aren't designed to scare you, though. I want to show you that you have a great opportunity to affect a small, responsive area of your body and bring about noticeable, positive changes elsewhere. We can help to ease knee arthritis simply by choosing the right footwear. We can prevent a multitude of lower limb problems by stretching one muscle group around the ankle. We may even be able to stop back pain... by massaging our feet!

In this chapter, you'll learn some techniques for preventing the common foot and ankle issues we help people with in my clinic. You'll also learn how to connect to your feet again, something we rapidly lose the ability to do in modern society. Pull your socks up and let's dip a toe into everything to do with the feet and ankles.

Stop Achilles Tendon Pain in Its Tracks

Do you remember classical history lessons at school? The legend of the great Greek warrior Achilles was one of my favourite stories to study.

The legend has it that at one point he was invincible; the greatest fighter ancient Greece had ever seen. His skill played a major part in the conquering of Troy, a so-called impenetrable city. The story goes that he was eventually felled in this battle by an arrow that struck him through his heel; the first significant - and ultimately catastrophic - injury anyone had inflicted on him across any of the battles he had fought.

The legend of Achilles has been preserved by the anatomy textbook authors, who have dubbed the large tendon that joins the calf muscle to the heel the *Achilles* tendon. You can find your Achilles tendon at the back of your calf, just above the heel, and it feels like a tough rope that you can easily grasp with two fingers. It is the largest tendon in the human body (a tendon joins muscle to bone) and it allows our calf muscles to pull on the heel and propel us onto our tiptoes.

However, a great many people suffer from a problem with the Achilles tendon which can do a very good job of stopping a usually active individual in their tracks[1]. Achilles tendon pain usually starts as a niggle felt in the tendon itself or immediately beneath it, right on the heel bone. It often flares up during the first few minutes of walking and in the morning, then settles as you get warm. In more severe cases, it can be painful literally all the time that you're on your feet and can significantly affect walking and running for many people.

We call Achilles tendon pain "*Achilles tendinopathy*" (you might have heard of the term "*Achilles tendinitis*" - which is an old fashioned term for exactly the same thing). This term basically means that there's a problem with the tendon or in the area that the tendon attaches to the bone. The problem can be either inflammation, tiny little tears in the tendon, or the tendon holding on to too much water. All of these issues lead to the same result: a nagging pain at the back of the heel.

Luckily, unlike the injury suffered by our old hero Achilles, this type of pain at the back of the heel is usually curable. If Achilles tendon pain has just started for you, our usual advice would be to rest for a couple of days and avoid any long walks or runs if at all possible. Usually, the pain will pass within three days.

However, if the pain has continued for longer than three days, a different approach is needed. Achilles tendon pain is usually preceded by a lack of strength in the calf muscles, which often goes undetected for many years, and can lead to excessive strain on the tendon[2]. When I say "*lack of strength*", what I'm really referring to is a lack of strength *in relation* to the demands you're asking of the tendon. For example, my Achilles tendon is strong enough for me to walk five miles or for me to work out in the gym for an hour without any bother at all, because I do those things regularly. However, if you asked me to run a marathon tomorrow, I'd be putting my Achilles tendon (and many other areas of my body) under intense pressure, something that it isn't used to.

This is a classic scenario for Achilles tendon pain. We often see it in people who go from being largely sedentary to suddenly deciding to take up an intense activity (we often call these people the "*weekend warriors*").

This is one of the dangers of deciding to start out on a workout programme like *"Couch to 5K"* (where the participants are encouraged to start running and build up rapidly to 5 kilometres of running distance). The Achilles tendon does not cope well with sudden changes in activity levels - and it may punish you for defying it.

A good general rule I tell my clients who are planning to increase their activity level is to only change one variable at a time (distance walked, duration of time walked or speed of walking) by a maximum of 10% at any one time. This is a great way to safeguard against Achilles tendon problems and many other injuries.

If you are already suffering from Achilles tendon pain, there are some steps you can take to reduce the pain and improve the health of the tendon that I'd like to share with you:

- **First of all, don't stretch the calves:** One of the common Achilles pain myths purported by runners, doctors and the general population alike is that if you have pain in your Achilles you should start stretching it out. A stretch that is commonly recommended is one where you place one foot behind the other while standing, then bend the front knee. Unfortunately, this stretch has not been shown to improve Achilles tendon problems and holding this position for a long time **may actually make the injury worse**, not better. Stretching the Achilles tendon can compress the injured part of the tendon and irritate the area, flaring it up and delaying healing[3]. While this effect doesn't occur for everyone, I think it is wise to resist the temptation to stretch the calf if you're suffering from this type of pain.

• **Wear supportive shoes with a heel:** For a short period of time, it is advisable to wear trainers and other shoes with a slight heel raise wherever possible[3]. This will lift your heel up and take any stretch away from the Achilles tendon, allowing it to heal better for the reasons stated in the point above.

• **Try to build some strength in your calves:** As one of the main causes of Achilles tendon problems is a mismatch between calf strength and the demands you're placing on the muscle, strengthening the calves can reverse the injury process and help the Achilles tendon to heal. There is a simple exercise you can do each day that will help to strengthen the calf muscles. Simply stand with your feet shoulder-width apart with something to hold onto. Then, raise yourself up onto your tiptoes before taking a slow count of four seconds to return to the floor (demonstrated opposite in figure A). Keep going with repetitions of this exercise until you feel some fatigue in your calf muscles. If you can do more than fifteen repetitions with ease, repeat this exercise but standing on just one leg.

• **Try to limit walking distance until it heals:** A lot of people choose to take the "*no pain, no gain*" approach when it comes to aches and pains. Unfortunately, more often than not, this isn't the right way forward and lands you in a worse situation than when you started. If the pain is continuing after the first fifteen minutes of your walk, don't simply try to push through the Achilles tendon discomfort. Pick a distance and pace that you can consistently walk at without setting off the pain and try to stick to it.

• **Use ice on the painful area to reduce soreness:** Using ice over the sore spot on the Achilles tendon can improve your symptoms and help to settle inflammation. It won't "fix" the problem, but you'll certainly feel better afterwards. As with all ice advice in this book, protect the skin and only apply for fifteen minutes at a time.

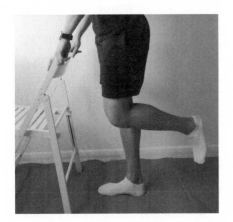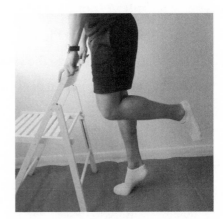

Figure A - Calf strengthening exercise

Fix Flat Feet & Improve Your Walking

It's likely that you've heard of the term "*flat feet*" before. Maybe someone - a physio or a podiatrist, most likely - even told you that you've got flat feet. But what does this funny term mean and why is it significant?

"Flat feet" (also called "*over-pronation*" or "*collapsed arches*") refers to a problem with the position that your feet are normally in when you're standing or walking. A normal foot posture consists of the front of the foot, the outside of the sole and the heel making contact with the ground as you stand still. A foot with good posture also has an arch, which should look almost like a cave on the inside of your foot when you're standing. The term "flat feet" refers to the **loss of that arch**. This means that the inside of the foot now also makes contact with the ground as well as the forefoot, outer sole and heel.

At this point, it is important to note that there is no "perfect" foot posture and there are plenty of normal, individual differences[4]. You only need to consider what footprints in the sand look like and how they differ from person to person, for instance.

However, with footprints within the range of "normal", you shouldn't be able to see the outline of the entire sole of the foot in the sand. You would see the heel, then a slim print of the outside of the sole, then the forefoot and toes. In someone with flat feet, you might see the entire sole making contact with the sand, which would make the footprints "fatter" in the middle.

But why do we care about flat feet, other than how our footprints might look on holiday?

The truth is, when you lose the arch in your foot and it becomes "flat", this alters the way the force travels through your foot and up into your leg when you walk. This means that the foot, ankle, knee and hip joints all have to compensate and adapt to this change in your mechanics.

Usually, our bodies are very clever and can adapt to these changes effectively; so effectively that we usually don't even notice. However, sometimes these adaptations can lead to problems over time. They can cause accelerated arthritis and stress on certain tissues in our ankles, knees, hips and even lower backs as a result[5]. This means that when someone finally realises there's a problem, it's often too late.

Some people believe that flat feet are a permanent, unsolvable problem. However, it's not quite as simple as that. It is true that flat feet are sometimes caused by the collapse of the ligaments that control our foot arch, and if this is the cause we can't do much about it except for wearing orthotics. In other cases, though, flat feet are just as a result of our foot muscles becoming "lazy" as a result of wearing supportive shoes too much of the time. These lazy foot muscles can lead to flat feet; with both of these features associated with lower limb pain[6].

I can give testament to this first-hand. When I worked in a hospital, my uniform policy allowed me to wear trainers at work as I often had to demonstrate exercises to my patients in the gym. Before I started at work, I invested in some expensive, super-comfortable, highly cushioned trainers that felt fantastic on my feet. When I walked, I felt like I was walking on air.

Several months passed and I went away for a long weekend on a walking holiday. I walked something like thirty miles in the three days I was away. I wore sturdy shoes suitable for walking, but they weren't the trainers I'd been wearing to work each day.

I came back from that holiday with plantar fasciitis (characterised by a searing pain in my heel) in not one but *both* feet, which lasted for about twelve weeks following that weekend. I couldn't understand how I'd developed this problem, seemingly out of the blue so suddenly. Then I looked at my feet, which have always historically been in good nick… and both my arches were as flat as a pancake.

Wearing my super-supportive trainers all day every day had effectively given my foot muscles a free ride. They had switched off, refusing to do any work. And they clearly continued to refuse even when I took my trainers off. So, when I went on my walking weekend, I had no foot strength to draw on and I developed this problem as a result. Lesson learned. I now only wear those trainers to play squash once a week.

If you've just looked down and realised your feet may be flat, my recommendation would be two-fold. First, I'd recommend that you try not to always wear the most supportive shoes you can find. As long as you don't have pain, try walking barefoot around the house and wearing sandals outside of the house in the summer rather than trainers. Try not to go for walks with dramatically built-up boots or padded heels. Let your feet do a bit of work for a change. It's the only way they'll get strong again.

My second recommendation would be for you to dedicate a bit of time to *reconnecting* with your foot muscles. Yes, this sounds like a very bizarre concept but hear me out. When our feet don't have to work as hard as they were designed to, we lose the ability to control the muscles within them. Have you ever seen someone with disabled upper limbs learn to paint using their feet with extraordinary skill and precision? Do you think they were born with this ability? Of course not. They put in the time to practice and can now connect to their feet.

Now, before you pick up a paintbrush with your toes and attempt to paint a grand Picasso replica, let's start with something a little simpler. Try the following exercise for several minutes each day, either underneath your table at your work desk or at home while watching TV:

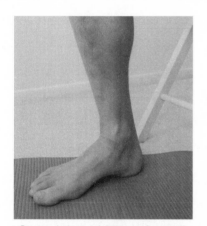 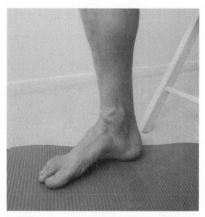

Start sitting with your foot relaxed on the floor. Keeping your toes and heel in contact with the floor at all times, use the muscles in your feet to lift your inner arch as high as you can. Hold for 2 or 3 seconds, then return to the relaxed position. Repeat 10-15 times in a row, whenever you get a quiet moment to sit.

How to Stop Twisting Your Ankle

"I keep twisting this damn ankle!" - Several years before I became a physio, I naively believed that I was the only one who suffered the frustration of multiple ankle sprains, always on the same side.

I used to put it down as being clumsy on one side; I am heavily right handed, after all. But when I started working and saw many people with the exact same issue as me - painfully rolling the same ankle every few weeks - I knew I wasn't alone.

It becomes a vicious cycle for many people. You twist your ankle, the ankle gets weak, you finally feel able to start walking on it… only to twist it again almost immediately and repeat the cycle, ad nauseum.

Does this sound familiar?

When I worked in professional sport, one of our key goals was to prevent this happening to the footballers we looked after. They would regularly sprain an ankle, often putting them in the physio room for 4-6 weeks at a time, and if that sprain became recurrent then it was catastrophic for the player and the team. So, we developed clever ways of rehabilitating these common sprains to stop them from happening over and over again.

If only I had known these clever tricks when I was a young lad spraining my ankle every 3 or 4 weeks, I could've avoided all that frustration too!

When you sprain your ankle, or any other joint in the body for that matter, you get three problems occurring all at once:

1. **The physical injury:** This refers to the damage to the ligaments (tough bands of tissue that hold your joints together) plus or minus strains to the surrounding muscles. Most ligaments and muscles heal up well over a period of several weeks, but some can remain damaged and that leads to an unstable joint if left to its own devices.

2. **Loss of muscle strength:** When your brain identifies damage somewhere in your body, one of the ways it protects your body from further damage is by *"shutting off"* the muscles around that joint temporarily. You may have experienced this after an ankle sprain; even though the bone wasn't broken, you probably struggled to put weight through your foot, as if the strength was completely gone. That is this loss of strength effect at work. The muscle strength does recover on its own over a few weeks to some degree but even when you feel strong again, there will still be weakness in some movements or actions[7].

3. **Loss of coordination - or "proprioception":** The term *"proprioception"* means your ability to tell what position your body is in without needing to look down and see. If you shut your eyes and you raise your arm up in front of you, you can tell that your arm is raised away from your side without needing to open your eyes. This is your internal proprioception system at work, and it's controlled by little receptors all over your body called *proprioceptors*. After you injure your ankle, your proprioceptors effectively malfunction and fail to work as well as they did before the twist (this is why ankle twists can

become recurrent)[7]. Without proper rehabilitation, your proprioceptors will continue to function poorly, putting you at risk of further injury.

These three problems all combine to cause a problematic ankle that twists or gives way regularly. The only way to avoid this is by reversing the damage to your ligaments, and loss to your strength and proprioception over a period of several weeks to months. I promise the hard work is worth it if you're able to avoid recurrent injuries for the rest of your life (plus avoid the risk of a more "serious" injury from a fall because of a dodgy ankle). Here are the three steps I encourage everyone with an ankle injury to take to prevent consequences later down the line:

1. **Let the joint heal!** Too many people, myself included, rush back into physical activity too soon following a sprain. By "physical activity", what I'm referring to is long walks, walking on rough terrain, exercise classes at the gym and running, among other things. All of these activities may *feel* alright at the time, but all it takes is a slight slip and you're back to square one. How long you avoid these things for is very individual and depends on how bad the initial injury was, so be sure to get advice for your own personal circumstances. You should certainly continue to try to weight-bear as early as you feel able, but do this through taking short walks and pottering around at home, not by taking intense "exercise".

2. **Rebuild muscle strength:** Of utmost importance is your effort in re-building any lost strength around your ankle. As every sprain is slightly

different, everyone has weakness in slightly different areas around their ankle, so some personalised recommendations are needed in each case. Book an appointment to see a physiotherapist with experience of dealing with ankle sprains for best results. However, building calf strength by trying to go up onto your tiptoes is a good place to start, as demonstrated on page 177.

3. **Re-train your proprioceptors:** As important as rebuilding your strength is rebuilding your proprioception. One important job of your proprioceptors is to allow you to balance. Therefore, any balance practice will also improve your proprioception. For rehabilitation, it's important to have a personalised programme as everyone will have different goals and needs, but try the exercises suggested in the "No Hands!" balance chapter of this book on page 147.

The most important thing to remember about ankle sprains is that just because the pain is gone from your ankle, it doesn't mean the problem has resolved. The structures may have healed well, but you're likely to still be suffering from a loss of strength and proprioception. Early action is key, as each subsequent sprain is harder to recover from. Don't delay, start taking the right steps early and ensure ankle longevity for many years to come!

Reconnect with Your Feet

When we were neanderthals, we didn't have the modern-day luxury of shoes. This meant that walking was always done barefoot. Our feet would've been toughened by hard callouses, resistant to jagged stones and hot ground.

Our feet would've been "internally" tough too. The muscles within our feet (all 20 of them) would've been strong and well-coordinated, able to propel us forward as we walked barefoot. Unfortunately, finding someone with feet like this is a rare occurrence in today's world.

Our supportive footwear and comfortable trainers feel great on our feet and allow us to walk and run without pain - but at a price. Over time, we've lost the robustness of our feet and the integrity of the subtle arches that give us proper foot function has suffered too. When our shoes provide protection and support, the muscles in our feet no longer need to work as hard as they once did. The old adage is that if you don't use it, you lose it; this applies to our foot muscles just as accurately as it does elsewhere.

The negative effects of a loss of foot muscle strength include increased risk of foot problems like plantar fasciitis, greater likelihood of knee and hip problems and possibly even an accelerated ageing process throughout the lower limbs[5,6]. You'll also be less efficient when walking and running, if these happen to be your hobbies.

So, what can be done to counter the effects of "lazy feet" caused by our modern footwear?

For a start, you can make an effort to not "over-wear" comfortable supportive footwear. Providing you don't have any pre-existing problems, it may be a good idea to make an effort to walk around the house barefoot as much as possible, or at least in flat, unsupportive slippers. Trainers are definitely still useful, but try to reserve them for just sporting activities.

If you're a lady who wears heels regularly, try to walk without heels where possible until a time when the occasion dictates that you absolutely need to wear them. I had a client who was making an effort to avoid heels because of an ankle problem but she had a fancy dinner party coming up the following weekend. I recommended that she wear flat shoes right up until she was about to get out of the car outside the dinner party, then put her heels on for the event, taking them off in the car again afterwards. It worked out that she only had to walk in heels from the car to the dinner table and back, rather than all the additional walking in heels had she worn them the entire evening from her house to the event.

Another solution I regularly recommend to my clients is to begin a foot strengthening regime. This may sound bizarre but it's actually quite simple to build such a thing into your routine.

I have covered my top recommended exercise for this purpose elsewhere in the book, but here's a recap of my favourite foot strengthening exercise: Start sitting, and place the edge of a towel under your toes. Using the muscles within your feet and toes (without letting your heel lift off the floor), grip the towel repeatedly as if to pull it towards you along the floor. Once you've scrunched the towel up entirely, roll the towel back out to its original position again and repeat (as demonstrated on page 126).

You'll notice as you perform this exercise that the natural arch on the inside of your foot has to lift to pull the towel in. This is good. It is being lifted by the muscles in your feet that may have been "switched off" for quite some time. Maintaining a good arch on the inside of your foot is an important safeguard against foot, knee and hip problems alike, and the more you practice this exercise the more permanent the change will become.

Fix Plantar Fascia Heel Pain in Three Simple Steps

As anyone who has suffered with plantar fascia heel pain can tell you, it really is a pain in the, well, foot.

As someone who has personally suffered with this problem (on both feet, no less) I can attest to the fact that it can be frustrating and even debilitating to some extent.

But what actually is plantar fasciitis and why is it so common?

In the underside of our feet, we have a tough band of fibrous tissue called the plantar fascia that joins the front of our foot to the heel. Without this band of tissue, our feet would be a shapeless mess, flat as a pancake, with no arch whatsoever. The plantar fascia is a very important part of our anatomy. If you think of a traditional long-bow (like the kind Robin Hood used once upon a time), the plantar fascia represents the bow string while the bow itself is the rest of the foot. If the bow string isn't present, the bow loses its tension and shape very quickly (as well as becoming effectively useless until re-strung). This is a metaphor that I like to use when talking about the plantar fascia.

You can feel your own plantar fascia by feeling along the underside of your foot from the heel, along the tough, fibrous, rope-like band in the inside of the arch, right up to the forefoot. This is the plantar fascia. The pain that occurs in this condition usually occurs right where the plantar fascia attaches to the heel. It can sometimes feel like the heel bone itself is painful. Pain can also often be felt inside the arch of the foot too. The layman's term for plantar fasciitis is "Policeman's heel", so-called because this heel pain can be caused by excessive walking (as your typical bobby might have to partake in while walking the beat).

The reason the plantar fascia can become problematic for some is largely due to the mechanics within our feet. When you walk, the job of the plantar fascia is to transmit force from your heel to your forefoot as you propel yourself forward. This job is usually shared by the plantar fascia and the muscles within the foot.

Pain can occur when you over-rely on the plantar fascia to do this job and neglect the other areas that are needed to perform this function.

This problem can be caused by a number of underlying issues, including but not limited to:

- **Tightness in the calves:** Because they attach to your heel, when your calves become tight they pull upwards on the heel which makes the entire operational "unit" of your lower leg and foot (calf, plantar fascia and foot muscles) tight, and changes the mechanics within the foot[8]. Don't worry too much about the specific mechanics involved, but remember that tight calves are almost always a bad thing.

- **Weakness in the foot muscles:** Refer to the previous section in this book where I talked about the reasons for foot muscle weakness and how it can cause problems.

- **Tightness within the plantar fascia itself:** While this is usually a secondary problem arising from one of the other causes, it is an issue

190

that still needs addressing. You can often feel if your plantar fascia is tight because it will be sore to the touch in your instep when you feel with your fingers as described earlier in this section.

- **Poor footwear selection:** Just to complicate matters, wearing either super-supportive OR under-supportive footwear can directly or indirectly trigger plantar fasciitis. I can attest to this myself. The key here is to change things up from time to time and never get stuck in one pair of shoes for an extended period of time.

- **An injury that caused a collapsed foot arch:** It is possible to injure your foot in such a way that it causes a loss of the natural arch on the inside of the foot. If this arch is lost, the way we use our feet changes dramatically and this can lead to plantar fasciitis.

- **Too little exercise, followed by too much exercise:** Our bodies hate sudden changes in activity levels and they often complain to let us know about it. A sudden change in the distance, duration or pace of your walking or running can trigger plantar fasciitis[9]. The reason this happens is because suddenly increasing your walking can expose underlying weakness or tightness and poor mechanics. When we challenge ourselves, our walking or running technique can often slip as we get tired and it is at this point that problems occur.

So, what can we do about an episode of plantar fasciitis? Well, the good news is that it does get better, provided you do the right things to help it. However, although plantar fasciitis is usually "self-limiting" (which means it'll go away on its own eventually), if we don't address the underlying problems that caused it in the first place, we're vulnerable to recurrences later down the line.

Here are the 3 important steps I recommend to my clients when it comes to resolving plantar fasciitis that you can start putting into action today. Remember, with all the exercises in this section it's important to get the all-clear from your doctor or physiotherapist before putting them into action to check that they're suitable for you and your personal circumstances.

1. **Self-massage for pain relief:** Arguably the least important of the 3 steps, but I feel this step can bring some value and certainly helped me when I was a sufferer. By taking a hard ball, like a golf or hockey ball, placing it under your foot when sitting and rolling out the hard "knots" on the underside of your mid-foot and arch, you can help to relieve some of the pressure on the plantar fascia and help your foot recover faster. **Important note:** *Do NOT roll over the heel bone itself with the hard ball as this will aggravate the problem.*

2. **Stretch the calves:** Tight calves make plantar fasciitis much more likely and are probably the leading contributors to the pain. It makes sense, then, that stretching your calf will take some of the pressure off the foot and improve your symptoms. There is a way of stretching your calves that I've found to be most effective, which I've included as a diagram below. Hold the stretch for a minimum of 30-seconds,

repeating every couple of hours.

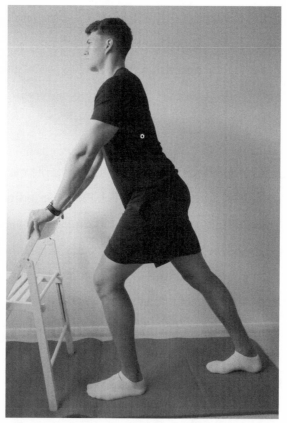

In this picture, the leg being stretched is the right leg. Put the leg to be stretched out behind you and assume the 'lunge' position shown in the picture. Feel free to lean on something in front of you. Keep your back heel down on the floor at all times. You should feel a stretch in your calf. Try to "lift" the arch on the inside of the foot that is being stretched if you can. Hold for 30-seconds, every 2-3 hours.

3. **Strengthen the foot again:** Through taking some time to strengthen the foot and the calf, over a period of time you can help your muscles to match up with the demands you're asking of them. The exercise in the *"Reconnect with Your Feet"* section on the previous pages is very effective here, as well as performing heel raises to fatigue several times each day, either standing on two or on one leg depending on your ability levels.

By putting into action these three steps, most people can expect their plantar fasciitis to resolve within a few weeks to several months in more persistent cases. The other important thing to do is to be assessed and advised by a physiotherapist who can identify any weak areas and mechanical problems that you may have missed in order to avoid this condition from coming back again, as it often can when not fully dealt with.

When to Use Orthotics

Orthotics are small inserts that go into your shoes with the purpose of lifting certain areas of your foot. They can be just big enough to cushion your heel, or they can raise up the entire foot to differing degrees. Some orthotics are firm while others are soft. You can get orthotics either off-the-shelf, or prescribed by a professional like a podiatrist.

So, in what circumstances are orthotics suitable?

This is a more complex question than it may originally seem. I've provided a list of problems that orthotics have helped some of my clients with, but it's impossible to guarantee they'll work for you too. I'd love to give you a list of injuries that orthotics *always* help with, but such a list unfortunately doesn't exist, mainly due to individual differences between you and your neighbour.

Let's first talk about how orthotics work and the potential problems we can run into through their use. Orthotics work by taking pressure away from a certain area of the foot and re-distributing it elsewhere. They can help to take a stretch off certain muscles, like the calves, and can almost instantly improve the symptoms of some conditions. They are useful in correcting subtle leg length discrepancies without necessitating the use of built-up orthopaedic shoes.

The problem is that reliance on orthotics for a long period of time can lead to semi-permanent changes to your movement mechanics[10]. Here's an example: imagine you feel a tightness in your calf when you walk, and you start to wear orthotics in your shoes. Upon introducing the orthotics, your symptoms disappear entirely as you've lifted your heel and thus taken the stretch off the calf muscle. However, you've removed the *symptom* by effectively placing the calf into an even shorter position (you just no longer feel the tightness as you've added some "slack" to the muscle with the orthotic) without addressing the *cause*. This means that, over time, your calf is going to adapt to this shortened position and become even tighter. Then, when removing the orthotic, your problem is much worse than it was when you began.

The same story is true when it comes to fixing "flat feet" or collapsed arches; you're artificially lifting the arch with the orthotic, which helps the *symptom* but actually worsens the underlying problem, further collapsing your arch in the long term.

The only way to tell if an orthotic is suitable for you is to consult a professional about your own individual circumstances. In my clinic, we provide a bespoke orthotic prescription service which will fit your feet with the right orthotic for the problem, as well as giving you advice on how to fix the problem over the long-term without the need for permanent reliance on the orthotic. We also never recommend orthotics to anyone who doesn't really need them - thus minimising unnecessary spending (and problems caused by over-wear of orthotics).

If you're wondering whether or not to try orthotics for your problem, be sure to seek advice from someone who offers a similar service to us. Navigating the world of orthotics alone can be difficult. Shop-bought orthotics can sometimes be effective; but there is such a range to choose from that the probability of making the wrong decision is very high.

Anyway, here is a list of complaints that some of our clients have found relief from by wearing orthotics as part of their treatment plan:

- Plantar fasciitis
- Achilles tendon pain
- Pain on the inside of the knee
- Pain on the side of the hip
- Bunions
- Arthritis of the ankle or big toe
- Recurrent ankle sprains
- Knee cap pain
- Lower back pain

If you're currently struggling with any of these problems, get in touch with us if you're local (we operate a no-improvement-no-fee policy) or find a local expert to help you decide whether it's worth pursuing a trial of orthotics.

The Problem with Tight Calves

This is something I touched on in some of the previous sections in this chapter, but it is a point worth driving home again and again.

Tight calves are not good. They are the origin and aggravator of many problems in the feet and ankles (and even elsewhere in the body). At one of the hospital systems where I once worked, they offered a "calf stretch class" dedicated to treating calf tightness, delivered to a class of 20 or more patients. For such significant financial outlay to have been authorised by the big-wigs in the hospital system, the specialists there must agree with me that addressing tight calves should be a priority.

The reason tight calves can be so problematic is because of the effects that they have on the other structures around the calf and foot. Some of the most common problems caused by tight calves are plantar fasciitis, Achilles tendon pain and pain at the back of the knee[11]. Calf pain can also be present, but, surprisingly, this often isn't a symptom.

Tight calves pull at their attachments on the heel bone and at the back of the knee, tugging other structures out of their intended position and stopping certain muscles from doing their intended job. They put stress on the Achilles and the plantar fascia in the foot, leading to an exponential increase in the likelihood of problems in these areas[12].

So, what can cause our calves to become tight?

There are probably a number of factors causing your calves to tighten up. One of them is definitely your choice of footwear. Wearing shoes with a heel puts the calf in a shortened position - and the body quickly adapts to the things we do often.

I also believe strongly that everyone should have a good stretch from time to time, and while most people over fifty are very good at remaining active, they are quite poor at following any exercise up with a good stretch afterwards!

The solution to a tight calf problem that I present to my clients at HT Physio consists of a combination of stretching and hands-on treatment. This two-pronged approach is vastly superior to just one or the other alone, in my opinion. The hands-on treatment helps to provide a rapid boost in the flexibility of the calf muscle, while the stretching done afterwards helps to maintain any gain in range of movement.

If you're a walker and you wish to continue walking for many years to come, I would recommend pre-empting calf problems and addressing any potential tightness long before a problem arises. I've seen people with calves so tight that they were beyond conservative treatment and had to undergo a "surgical release" of the muscle to treat the problem. Avoiding surgery is always better than having to go under the knife, and early action is the key.

A great gentle stretch you can try at home to treat tight calves, provided you get the all-clear for your particular circumstances before you try it, is demonstrated on page 193.

Which Shoes are Right for Me?

As this is something I am frequently asked about, I wanted to dedicate a short section of this book to choosing the right shoes for some of the common situations we all face each day. I've mentioned footwear a few times in this chapter and I understand it can be confusing when it comes to choosing the right option. Should you opt for the most comfortable? Or do you go for flat, sturdy, "sensible" shoes? This section has the answers.

I must preface this section by reminding you that everyone is different, so you should disregard my recommendations if you have a painful problem that is aggravated by changing your shoes, or you get contradictory advice from another healthcare professional.

For long walks: I always recommend to people that they opt for walking boots with a built-up ankle to protect against sprains and twists. Walking boots are designed to be durable and protective over long distances, so if walking is your main hobby then they are worth the investment. In general, opt for the ones that are most comfortable in the shop as long as they support the ankle area as well as the foot.

For daily wear: I recommend wearing a variety of shoes for day-to-day wear. Mix it up between trainers, flat shoes and, if you are female, heels, if these are to your taste. I advise regularly changing shoes day-to-day so that your feet and lower limbs don't adapt too much to any one pair of shoes, as this can become problematic.

For evening wear: Taking fashion into account, I'm absolutely unopposed to people wearing whatever they like in the evenings, provided they are comfortable and a pre-existing painful problem isn't flared up by their choice.

For the gym or running: Opt for sturdy running shoes with a firm sole. There are a huge variety of running shoes on the market and a lot of them have flimsy soles that you can quite easily bend and twist. Here's the rule: If you can bend the shoe in half, it's probably not protective enough for running. With trainers, you generally get what you pay for in terms of durability and protection, but a recent study in the British Journal of Sports Medicine interestingly did not show a correlation between money spent and effectiveness of running shoe[13].

CHAPTER SEVEN

Whole-Body Health

Introduction

So far, we've covered each area of your body separately in this book, hopefully giving you strategies for ensuring your joints and muscles stay healthy and injury-free. However, if I was to conclude the book here, I'd be making an enormous oversight.

You see, our bodies aren't just a collection of different muscles and joints that just so happen to work together. We, as humans, are much more than that. We operate as one whole, complex organism, not just a sum of our parts. Therefore, from this point on, we're going to be thinking about our bodies as one magnificent ecosystem; that thrives through a complex plethora of chemical reactions and processes happening inside of us every single minute.

By making small yet significant decisions on the way we live our lives, we can influence these complex processes and ensure the entire body benefits. In this chapter, we're going to discuss how to limit harmful inflammation, how to improve your hormone profile (which governs over the entirety of your health and wellbeing), and even how to stave off bone fragility in old age. Once we stop seeing ourselves as just a sum of our body parts and start realising how even the smallest changes can affect the rest of us through a cascade of reactions, amazing things can happen.

The Problem with Inflammation (& Do I Have It?)

Inflammation has become one of those common buzzwords that strikes fear into those who hear it in the context of heath.

Inflammation refers to a natural process in the body whereby certain chemicals are released by damaged or injured cells, causing the surrounding blood vessels to leak fluid into nearby tissues, often causing swelling. Reading that passage, it does sound like inflammation is a bad thing; but that would be far too simplistic a view of this complex process.

Inflammation isn't always a process to be feared or avoided. When we exercise, for example, our muscles undergo damage which leads to inflammation. It is this damage, and the consequential recovery process that occurs directly afterwards, that causes our muscles to grow and become stronger.

In another common situation, such as when we sprain or strain a joint within the body, the first helpful step of the healing process is inflammation[1]. The swelling that appears around a joint after you injure yourself is part of the body's plan to clear that area of debris and waste, allowing proper healing to occur. So, in many cases, inflammation isn't "bad" or something we necessarily want to avoid.

However, there are obviously times when inflammation can be harmful to us. One of such times is during the process of "global inflammation", which basically means there are high levels of inflammatory chemicals in the bloodstream. The problem with global inflammation is that it can lead to tissue damage in many areas within the body, weight gain[2], and generally feeling pretty terrible. However, one of the main additional reasons I like to educate my clients on inflammation is because of the detrimental effects global inflammation can have on *healing* from injury.

Some of the signs of global inflammation are multiple joint pains, puffy areas on your body (especially the face) and difficulty losing weight (or more weight gain than usual). If you have any of these symptoms, I would recommend a trip to the doctor's for a routine blood screen which can help to identify the cause of the symptoms.

Global inflammation can be caused by several diseases or chronic conditions (which are well beyond the scope of this book) but it can also be caused by our daily choices and habits. The choices we make every day impact the delicate chemical balance in our bloodstreams profoundly.

As an obvious example, choosing to eat tonnes of sugary food for breakfast, lunch and dinner can significantly drive up global inflammation in our bodies and even lead to problems like diabetes[3]. While most people know to avoid lots of sugar, there are other less obvious choices and habits that can also have an effect on inflammation.

Some of the "hidden" foods that have been shown to cause inflammation include certain types of vegetable and seed oils, which are often added to our foods unknowingly. Foods that are "ready-made" in stores or in many restaurants are regularly prepared with excessive amounts of these harmful oils and can worsen inflammation.

Processed meats and "junk food" with high levels of trans fat have also been proven to accelerate inflammation[4]. I always recommend to my clients that they opt for supermarket or butcher's meat with as little processing between it being a living animal and on your plate. I'm also an advocate for free-range and organic meats where possible, but the high cost involved can often deter people. Instead, a good approach can be to choose your most common meat products from the free-range and organic section. For me, I opt for free-range eggs from organic chickens as I eat eggs every morning. I also buy my chicken free-range and organic but the meats I eat less often, like beef, I buy in the regular range from the supermarket, simply due to cost. You may choose to purchase foods differently based on your budgetary, dietary and ethical choices. The important thing is finding a healthy plan that works for you and that you can stick to.

Two major causes of global inflammation are smoking and drinking. We all know about the detrimental effect to your lungs from smoking, but smoking also drives up inflammatory chemicals in the bloodstream and can dramatically slow down the healing process from almost any injury[5]. My friendly advice to you, should you be a smoker, would be to seek an alternative with a view to weaning yourself from tobacco. There are some fantastic innovations available at the moment in terms of patches and gum which can help you stop smoking, as well as most health centres offering free smoking cessation advice.

The other perspective to take on smoking is to analyse yourself from a behavioural point of view. Many smokers are less "chemically addicted" than they might seem but highly "behaviourally addicted"[6]. This means that they associate having a cigarette with relief from a negative emotion, like stress. Getting help for something like this is well beyond the scope of this book, but I just want to make you aware that there is help available to change these cognitive-behavioural patterns.

Drinking heavily is also a common cause of global inflammation[7]. One of the causes of the classic "beer belly" seen in regular heavy drinkers is actually inflammation. Inflammatory chemicals in the blood send a trigger to the body to store fat around the mid-riff and our internal organs[8]. This is obviously not a good thing, and not just because of the appearance of a large beer belly. While I am certainly not against a drink from time to time, if you have a regular drinking habit you'd probably benefit from cutting down some. There are also resources available for people looking to cut down on drinking, so if you have found your alcohol units each week creeping up over time, it may be worth seeking out some information locally.

If you do have inflammation, the best way to relieve it is by making positive changes to your diet and lifestyle. As I'm not a dietician, I cannot make specific recommendations to you about which foods you can or cannot include in your diet, but I'll share with you some of the facts about foods which have been reported to help with reducing inflammation.

One of such families of food is green leafy vegetables, like kale and broccoli. These wonderful greens can help to improve the longevity of healthy cells in the human body and can reduce inflammation, as well as providing fibre and other nutrients that are positive to health[9].

We talked about vegetable oils often being a poor choice earlier, but did you know that coconut and olive oil have been shown to have the opposite effect on inflammation[10,11]? The research shows that coconut and olive oil has anti-inflammatory effects, so making that substitute to your cooking may be advisable. Don't go crazy with the oils though; remember that these "healthy" oils are still highly calorific, and being overweight does result in increased global inflammation.

The healthy fats in certain nuts, like walnuts, and in oily fish, like mackerel and salmon, can also help to drive down inflammation[12]. The government health authorities recommend that we include two portions of oily fish in our diet every week[13]. Are you getting yours?

Berries are another proven anti-inflammatory superfood. Blueberries and raspberries are great choices to include in breakfast and as snacks due to their anti-oxidant properties, helping to cut inflammation[14].

While these foods have all been shown to encourage a reduction in inflammation in the body, it's important to also address diet as a whole to get any positive effects whatsoever. It's no good adding a few berries in with your breakfast then continuing to eat junk food for the rest of the day and still expecting a positive effect! Most of the people I serve understand this already, and are able to make just a few small tweaks to their diet to bring about a positive effect.

My final point on this subject will be to tell you one more thing that does improve global inflammation in almost every case: general exercise. Taking several brisk walks every week can improve health in many respects[15], and the effects it has on global inflammation are no different. Keep active, eat well, make good choices and inflammation shouldn't be your enemy any longer!

Improve Your Hormones (For Over 50's)

Although I'm not a doctor or a hormone specialist, I do speak with many patients over fifty each and every day who are suffering from problems associated with changing hormones.

Some of the common problems my clients report to me include high cholesterol (which can put you at risk of heart disease), inflammation, weight gain, urinary leakage, loss of sexual desire and even memory problems - all of which can often be linked to fluctuations in hormones as we age.

If you're suffering with hormonal symptoms like the ones listed above, the first thing to realise is that you're definitely not alone! These problems are extremely common, and while that doesn't make them any more pleasant to deal with, it can provide some comfort to know that you aren't going through this alone.

All of the above problems that I mentioned should ideally be discussed with your doctor to get some personalised advice about solutions that may be best for you. There are medications available that can control some of these unpleasant symptoms, so it's always worth having a chat with your GP about these issues.

However, it is also true that changes in your hormones can be partially as a result of lifestyle choices - good or bad. For example, high cholesterol and inflammation (which can wreak havoc with your hormones) can be helped greatly through committing to regular exercise and a diet low in sugar[3]. Eating plenty of fruit, vegetables, nuts and fish can also help. All of these changes contribute to cutting away belly fat, which is our enemy when it comes to unpleasant hormonal changes. The fat that we store around our midriffs produces inflammatory chemicals which can negatively affect our hormones and bring about many of the symptoms associated with the menopause[16].

Many women suffer from urinary leakage over fifty. Although extremely common, this unfortunately brings a lot of embarrassment for the women I help who have mentioned this me. It's upsetting to hear about the loss of confidence that many people suffer because of this issue, so I wanted to make everyone reading this aware of the fact that there is often a solution to this problem!

The muscles that control the flow of urine from the bladder are called the "pelvic floor", and like any other muscle group, it can become weak and unable to do the job it was designed for. Luckily, as we've discussed many times in this book already, muscles can be effectively strengthened and the pelvic floor is no different! The research supports this fact, too. A recent systematic review on the topic found that pelvic floor strengthening exercises were 17 times as effective in treating urinary incontinence as no treatment[17].

The exercises needed to do this job are quite simple and can be done anywhere at any time of the day, but they do require some supervision to get started and to make sure you're doing them correctly. If you're suffering from this problem, I would recommend searching for a women's health physiotherapist in your area and getting some instruction on how to strengthen your pelvic floor muscles.

One of the most common hormonal problems for men as we age is a loss of testosterone. Research has shown that men's testosterone levels decline by about 1% every year after age forty[18]! Low testosterone has been linked to loss of sexual desire, erectile dysfunction, muscle loss and even depression[19].

All of these symptoms should be investigated by a doctor, but there are a few common causes for low testosterone that should definitely be addressed too. For a start, low vitamin D levels have been associated with decreased testosterone. Luckily, research has shown that vitamin D supplementation may help to normalise testosterone again[20]. Some experts even recommend that everyone starts taking a vitamin D supplement, especially those over fifty (and people in colder climates). This recommendation is due to the fact that our skin becomes less efficient at absorbing vitamin D from the sunlight as we age, so we must strive to get it from other sources[21].

On the topic of vitamin D, there is even research to show that being deficient can seriously increase your risk of dementia. In a University of Exeter study, adults aged sixty-five or older who were moderately deficient in vitamin D had a 53 percent higher risk of developing dementia; for the severely deficient, the risk rose to 125 percent[22].

Another contributor to a loss of testosterone in ageing men is a lack of physical exercise, especially resistance training. The benefits of resistance training are too great to ignore, which is why there is a section of this book dedicated solely to resistance training for over-50's (and a free gift for you at the back of this book). One of these benefits is a significant increase in serum testosterone levels following a period of weight training, as seen in a study in the Journal of Applied Physiology[23].

Exercising against resistance, which I'd argue is one of the best things you can do for your body, can help to cut fat, improve strength and balance your hormones, as well as maintain mobility[24]. I usually recommend that people try to include exercises called *compound movements* in their regime as much as possible. Compound movements involve more than one joint and muscle group working at the same time. Squatting, picking something up from the floor or standing up from a chair are great examples of compound movements that strengthen more than one area of the body.

Many of the exercises I've recommended in this book constitute compound movements but for a regime that is personalised to your needs, it's always best to get individual advice from a physiotherapist or a personal trainer who is qualified in exercise prescribing.

Resistance training is equally as important for women suffering from hormonal fluctuations as well, and can stave off osteoporosis[25] (or thinning of the bones) which is more common in post-menopausal women (more on that in the next chapter).

Overall, it's important to remember that you aren't helpless to the changes occurring in your body as you age, and there are practical solutions available to combat the effects of ageing. You've got a lot of living to do yet, so let's make sure those years are happy, healthy and fulfilling!

Combating Osteoporosis

Often confused with osteoarthritis, *osteoporosis* is actually a separate condition entirely. Osteoporosis is a condition where the bones in the body have thinned and become structurally weaker, leaving the victim vulnerable to fractures. The main contributing causes of osteoporosis include hormonal fluctuations, poor diet and a lack of physical exercise[26]. Notice how each of these three factors are within our control to some extent, which makes osteoporosis avoidable in many cases.

Unfortunately, osteoporosis is a very common problem for people over the age of fifty and it has a tendency to affect women more than men[27]. The reason women are more frequently affected tends to be due to the hormonal changes that occur during the menopause. Loss of oestrogen occurring during the menopause has been directly linked to osteoporosis and loss of bone mass[28].

Osteoporosis literally means "*porous bones*", which describes the appearance of affected bones when closely examined. There are certain areas that tend to be affected worse than others; these areas include the spine, hip and shoulder[27]. These also tend to be the areas that can become injured easily following even mild trauma after the start of osteoporosis, so avoiding this condition should be of paramount importance in order to preserve and ensure a long, active life.

So, what can we do to ward off osteoporosis as we get older?

There are bone scans, often called DEXA scans, which are effective at picking up bone thinning and can diagnose osteoporosis (or *osteopenia - which is the earlier stage of osteoporosis). A good first step is to get your bone density tested if you have any concerns, just to know where you stand currently. If you know your starting point, it's easier to make a plan. If you've had a recent fracture and you are over the age of fifty, your doctor will usually send you for a DEXA scan as part of the follow-up process to check you haven't developed osteoporosis.

There are medications available for people who have developed osteoporosis, which correct deficiencies in certain minerals and help to strengthen the bones again. However, prevention is always better than cure and if you can do it naturally, even better.

One way to ensure that you protect against osteoporosis is to make sure your diet is working in your favour to keep those bones strong. The body uses calcium and vitamin D as "building blocks" for bone, so ensuring that you include plenty of calcium and vitamin D in your diet is very important[29]. You can get calcium from dairy sources and meat, and vitamin D can be derived from sunlight as well as eggs and oily fish. If you lead a vegetarian or vegan lifestyle, you will have to take extra care to ensure you're getting enough of these vital nutrients and a supplement may be beneficial. Speak to your doctor or a nutritionist if you're unsure.

Another incredibly important factor in keeping bone loss at bay is physical exercise. While walking and remaining generally active are good for this purpose to an extent, there is one type of exercise that trumps them all when it comes to keeping the bones strong and healthy. This type of exercise is resistance training.

Resistance training is the process of pushing or pulling against the resistance of weights, your body weight or resistance bands. We've long known about the positive effects of resistance training on the muscles but it wasn't until relatively recently that more attention was given to the effects of resistance training on our bones. Through multiple studies, it's been proven that our bones strengthen as a direct response to resistance training[25]. This type of exercise increases our bone mass and can directly prevent osteoporosis. It's our body's way of saying *"If we're going to be lifting these weights from now on, I'm going to need good, strong bones to be able to do so!"*

As I mentioned in the hormone section of this book in the preceding pages, compound movements are again superior to "single joint" movements. Most of the actions you perform each day (like climbing the stairs or getting up from a chair) are all compound movements, involving movement of multiple joints in your body. These exercises have been shown to strengthen the bones more than single-joint movements.

To get an idea of which exercises I consider the best and often recommend to my over-fifty clients for optimal bone and muscle health, you can download my guide on *"The Top 5 Exercises for Over-50's Who Want to Remain Strong, Mobile & Active"* which is a free downloadable bonus for readers of this book. You can find it at: **ht-physio.co.uk/guide/**

Resistance Training Over Fifty

The last chapter brings us nicely onto one of the most important sections of this book - where I'm going to teach you a bit about what I consider to be the most important type of exercise that can possibly be considered for over-fifties.

Resistance training is the process of pushing or pulling against an external resistance, your body weight or resistance bands. There is huge variety in terms of exercises and movements to choose from when it comes to resistance training. You can strengthen almost any part of your body with some form of resistance training and as a general rule, the stronger you are, the healthier you are[30]. Resistance training also doesn't have to take much of your time to be highly effective. As little as 10-15 minutes done regularly can have a noticeable effect and is one of the principles I've used to change the lives of many clients in my business.

Long gone are the days when resistance training was just considered the realm of body builders and professional athletes. In fact, when asked by an older gentleman whether or not he was too old to start lifting weights, Arnold Schwarzenneger, arguably the greatest professional body builder of all time, said *"You are too old NOT to start lifting weights!"*

And he's absolutely right. The benefits of resistance training are too numerous and impressive to be overlooked by anyone who wants to remain active, mobile and as comfortable as possible throughout their advancing years. I should also mention that resistance training can genuinely add not just years, but *quality* years to your life.

Don't just take my word for it. Here are some of the proven positive effects of resistance training for over-fifties (referenced with scientific studies to support each claim) so you can decide for yourself:

• Resistance training will improve muscle strength and reduce your risk of injury as a result[31].

• It will improve joint and muscle flexibility and mobility[32].

• You'll lose body fat, but you'll also find it easier to keep the fat off as you gain muscle. Having more muscle on your body raises your metabolism meaning you burn more calories at rest than someone who is the same age as you but doesn't resistance train[33].

• There is some evidence to suggest that resistance training slows down cognitive decline in older adults[34].

• Your stamina will improve, meaning you won't get so tired when out walking with friends[35].

• Back pain can be treated through resistance training[36].

• You'll have a lower risk of anxiety and other mental health problems[37].

• Resistance training is a great way to protect against and treat arthritis[37].

• Your mobility and balance will improve, making falls less likely[31].

• You'll generally look better, as well as maintaining a younger-looking posture too[38].

• You'll have a lower risk of osteoporosis as your body lays down bone to cope with the demands of your resistance training[25].

• You'll get the wonderful side effects of improved confidence, self-esteem and body image, which may translate to improved libido and happiness[37].

• Your sleep should improve, meaning you can get off to sleep faster and with less disturbances through the night[37].

• You'll find that daily tasks become a breeze; no more heavy breathing when you get to the top of the stairs[38]!

• Resistance training has been shown to have positive effects on your heart and lungs, similar to those of cardiovascular training, meaning if you're going to prioritise one form of training, it should ideally be resistance work[38].

Such overwhelming evidence for taking up or continuing resistance training shouldn't be ignored and I'd encourage everyone reading this to get started, provided they are healthy enough to do so and there's no medical reason why they shouldn't. Of course, always get the all-clear from your doctor before starting any new regime.

So, how does one actually go about starting a resistance training regime?

You don't necessarily need to go and join a gym, although that would be a good idea if you've got one nearby that's easily accessible and within your budget. The benefits of joining a gym include access to safe, ready-to-use equipment and guidance from the staff should you need it. However, you can just as easily start some resistance training from the comfort of your own home with minimal equipment.

For readers of this book, I've created a valuable report titled "*The Top 5 Exercises for Over-50's Who Want to Remain Strong, Mobile & Healthy*" which I've made available as a free gift for you to download, as a thank you for reading this book. It'll give you the five best resistance exercises for over-fifties, and everything you need to keep you strong, mobile and healthy. All of these exercises can be done at home with only minimal equipment. These exercises will give you the most "bang for your buck", giving you the greatest strength and health benefits in the shortest time possible.

As a reader of this book, you can download it free by visiting:

ht-physio.co.uk/guide/

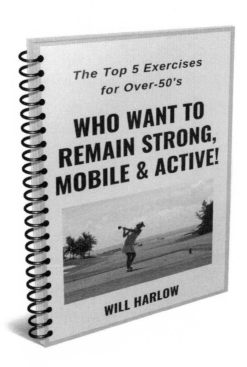

Overcoming a Broken Bone

Unfortunately, fractures and breaks (these terms mean the same thing and are used inter-changeably) can be life-changing; creating temporary or permanent disability on a physical level and severely knocking the confidence of the victim on an emotional level. If you've ever experienced a fracture, you'll know how much of an ordeal it can be. From the initial trauma, to the hospital waiting room, to the scans and x-rays, to the stiffness and discomfort, even to the downright cruel physiotherapist asking you to move that painful joint a week or two afterwards!

However, if you've recently suffered a break, there are some important principles to know which, when applied, will give you the best chance of recovery without on-going problems.

In general, broken bones need a period of no movement, called "immobilisation". What this period of time does is allows the bone to "re-set" to its original position. To allow this to happen, the body will start to lay down new bone over the area of the break. Just as a builder might begin by erecting scaffolding before laying down new bricks on a damaged house, the body operates in the same way. The new bone (scaffolding) laid down by the body is fragile and tender, so needs a certain period of time to harden up into "mature" bone (bricks).

It's important to say that the circumstances around every broken bone are different. This is why anyone who's broken a bone should be assessed by an orthopaedic consultant who can decide on the best management plan for their individual circumstances. Some fractures need as long as 8 weeks of no movement, while others can get going after 2 weeks. It's impossible for a non-medical person to make this decision safely for themselves, so be sure to always follow the guidance of your consultant.

After a period of no movement, it's then imperative that we start moving the injured area again. Movement sends a signal to the body that says we do indeed still need strong bones in that area. If you were to fracture a leg and then not move it for a whole year, the body would interpret that as a signal saying *"great, we don't need strong bones there anymore,"* and would, as a result, give up on properly healing the fracture; as well as taking away density of the surrounding bone too. Neither of those effects would do us much good.

This is why you might meet a cruel physiotherapist trying to move your arm or leg when you *really* don't want to! Although it doesn't feel like it very much at the time, it is certainly in your best interests.

Another important thing to understand is that starting to bear weight through a broken bone (after the initial "rest" period) is another way of telling the body that it needs to accelerate the healing process. This is especially true when it comes to lower limb fractures, such as a broken ankle.

If someone with an ankle fracture was to avoid putting weight on the ankle even when it was safe to do so, while another person with an identical injury chose to start trying to gently walk on that leg once safe, the person who made the effort to walk on the injured ankle would get back to normal far sooner. The body is an *adaptation* machine; it will respond to anything we throw at it. If we're asking it to walk on an injured bone, the body will make every effort it can to heal that bone, and consequentially allow us to walk again.

Now that we've covered the basics, is there anything else we can do to encourage a broken bone to heal faster?

The answer is: definitely. Small changes to your diet have been shown to accelerate fracture healing, such as ensuring you're getting enough calcium and vitamin D. Dairy and red meat will help with your calcium intake, and if you're vegan, look to green leafy vegetables, nuts and soy. The body creates vitamin D following exposure to the sunlight, so even though you may be injured, try to get yourself out the house if you can.

One very important factor helping you return to the things you love as soon as possible is ensuring the health of the unaffected joints and muscles around the broken bone. I could tell you many stories about patients who have fallen and broken their shoulder, but when they first came to see me it was actually their *elbow* that was giving them more bother. This tends to be very common with breaks in the upper limbs, as you'll often be put in a sling and told to "not move it" for a month or two. While that's all well and good for the broken bone trying to heal, the other parts of the arm also get immobilised - becoming incredibly stiff and painful as a result.

The only way to counteract this is to firstly be aware that stiffness will rapidly set in if you don't move these other healthy joints. That's why, in my example given about a broken shoulder, it's very important to still try and move the fingers, wrist and elbow each day (as long as your consultant is happy for you to do so) in order to keep these healthy areas mobile and minimise loss of muscle mass and strength.

The same is true of fractures in the lower limbs, too. I've seen many patients losing almost all of their thigh muscles after they've broken their ankle, simply because they are unable to walk and haven't used their thigh muscles in weeks. When I worked in professional football, when we had a broken bone in one of our players, our primary job in the early stages was to minimise muscle loss in other areas of the body while the injured bone healed. That often meant two or three hours in the gym each day, working on the muscles above and below the injured area. By doing this, when the plaster came off we were only dealing with one problem area, rather than three or four. This helped them get back on the pitch faster after the injury, which was a great result for the player (and the manager).

Unfortunately, in my experience many people over fifty are left to their own devices for a few weeks following a broken bone, before getting only a couple of physiotherapy sessions on the NHS. While they are given enough treatment to walk again, there are often still huge deficits in their strength, mobility - and even independence - compared to how they were before the injury. It's important not to just "accept" that things can never be the same following a fracture, especially if you haven't had thorough, in-depth treatment. At my clinic, we can often help people improve far beyond what they considered possible after being discharged from a big hospital system; so, if you're not satisfied with your results, I'd certainly recommend seeking out a second opinion.

The Truth About Glucosamine

Chances are, you know someone who is currently taking glucosamine for joint pain. Widely available from chemists and health food stores alike, glucosamine supplementation has really exploded in popularity over the last few years. But what *is* all the fuss about when it comes to glucosamine?

Glucosamine is a natural substance found in your cartilage, which helps to make up the layers of cushioning between your joints. It was hypothesised that taking glucosamine as a supplement can help to regenerate the cartilage within joints that are affected by arthritis, reducing joint pain as a result.

However, it turns out that this mechanism has never been conclusively backed up by science. There have been multiple studies done on the effects of glucosamine in joint pain from arthritis, and the results have been inconsistent to say the least. The largest study done on glucosamine supplementation for hip and knee pain showed no significant improvement in the symptoms of their participants over a period of six months[39]. Due to the results of this study, NHS workers are not supposed to formally recommend glucosamine to patients for joint health.

However, there have also been studies that have shown small improvements in symptoms of hip and knee arthritis after glucosamine supplementation[40]. Why the results of these studies differ is unclear. Some researchers have hypothesised that the type and dose of the supplement may be the key difference, while others have just said the differences have been down to sheer luck.

Either way, it's important to note that glucosamine supplementation (or any other supplementation for that matter) isn't without its risks. Glucosamine may interfere with warfarin; so, if you're taking a blood thinner you may want to reconsider self-medication with glucosamine. Glucosamine may also affect the way that the body reacts to sugar which may have implications for those with diabetes. The research also suggests that pregnant and breastfeeding women should probably avoid glucosamine (due to the lack of sufficient evidence around its safety during these sensitive times).

Anecdotally, I have heard of some clients who feel they have benefitted greatly from glucosamine supplementation, but for every one who has told me it worked for them, there is someone else who noticed no effect at all. If you're considering starting to supplement with glucosamine, it's advisable to talk to your doctor before you begin as there may be a reason why glucosamine is not a good solution for you.

Unfortunately, there is no magic pill for arthritis and the jury remains out when it comes to glucosamine. However, there are other things you can do to help, as I've mentioned many times in this book. Getting a targeted exercise regime to strengthen and mobilise your painful areas can significantly improve symptoms. So too can making good lifestyle choices whenever you can. The important thing to remember is that it's always worth seeking out an opinion, or a second opinion, on what can be done for your painful problem - oftentimes, help is available if you look for it.

The Science of Sleep

Do you remember when you were 18 or 19 years old and all you wanted to do was sit up all night?

For most people, entering working life puts an end to that desire to stay up every night as early mornings become a cruel necessity. We learn pretty quickly that when you get very little sleep, you function poorly the next day.

But why, on a scientific level, is sleep so important? Do we really need eight hours each night? And what happens to our health if we chronically allow our bodies less sleep than we need?

To answer these questions, I turned to information from prominent neuroscientist and sleep expert, Matt Walker, who is widely published online and has written a fantastic book of his own, called *Why We Sleep*[41].

Matt Walker has concluded from his research at the University of Berkeley, California, that anything less than seven hours of sleep constitutes sleep deprivation. And with sleep deprivation comes an increased risk of a multitude of health problems, including Alzheimer's Disease, cancer, diabetes, obesity and poor mental health.

Mr Walker also points out how badly we erode our sleeping hours in modern day society: going from 92% of people getting over six hours of sleep per night in 1942, to only 50% of people reporting six hours of sleep a night in 2017. The problem with this fact is that after just one night of less than five hours sleep, numbers of key immune cells (the ones that fight cancer) in our blood drop by up to 70%. This leaves us wide open to serious medical problems. Walker also squashes the myth that older adults need less sleep, and explains that getting sufficient sleep is an important factor in staving off the onset of dementia in many cases.

His work provides us with one of the most fascinating explanations for how sleep replenishes us that I've ever come across. In a related podcast with presenter Jordan Harbinger (*The Jordan Harbinger Show*), Walker explains how a substance called adenosine builds up in our brains during our waking hours. A high concentration of adenosine building up in the receptors in our brain causes us to feel tired. Walker calls this "sleep pressure". When we sleep, it's like "releasing the valve" and letting this pressure hiss away as the brain clears adenosine from its receptors.

Unfortunately, many people suffer from sleep problems or poor "sleep hygiene". If this sounds like you, there are certainly some steps you can take to improve your sleep without needing to reach for the sleeping pills.

For a start, most experts recommend that we set aside some time in the evening to wind down before bed, usually between thirty minutes and an hour (but possibly longer). During this time, lights should be dimmed, electronics (including the TV) should be switched off and voices in your household should be muted as much as possible. The effects from blue light emitted by phones and televisions have been well documented; they delay the process of falling to sleep, as well as preventing deep sleep[42].

Be sure to turn off all lights in your room before sleep, and I'm not just talking about your bedside lamp. Even the tiniest light in your room has the potential to disturb depth of sleep. That includes the numbers on your alarm clock, the standby light on the TV and even the blinking light on a smoke detector. One of the greatest investments I made a year or so ago was to purchase a set of black-out blinds for my room which cancel out the light from the streetlamp outside my bedroom window. I almost immediately noticed an improvement in my sleep.

It has also been documented that the best sleep occurs when your body temperature has dropped by about 1°C compared to that of waking[43]. This means it is important to keep a cool room at night. Surprisingly, having a hot bath before bed may also help. This is because the hot bath causes the blood vessels near the surface of our skin to dilate and the heat from our core to rise towards the surface and dissipate, cooling us off in the long run.

Finally, limiting coffee and caffeine after midday is also a strategy that Walker recommends. He chooses to go for such an early coffee-curfew because of the long half-life that caffeine has - which is around six hours. This means that, in a healthy adult, it takes around six hours for the body to clear *half* of the caffeine that we've ingested. This means that even a late morning coffee may still be active in your bloodstream by the time it comes to winding down for bed ten or more hours later.

From my own point of view and experience, I've found that people who get sufficient sleep tend to recover from injury faster than those who report disturbed or inconsistent sleep. The reverse is also true, and many of the patients I help with chronic conditions tend to be very poor sleepers. Based on this and the ever-growing body of research from scientists like Matt Walker, I would certainly recommend prioritising sleep high on your list along with diet and exercise if living a long, healthy life is your goal.

The Importance of a Healthy Weight

In 10,000BC, when the earliest humans walked the earth, food was scarce. Our ancestors would hunt for food - sometimes unsuccessfully - and when they made a kill, every precious morsel would be eaten or put to use in some way. Food was sacred, valuable and required our ancestors to put their lives in danger each time they ventured out to look for it.

Fast forward all these millennia and our circumstances have changed quite a bit. Food is now readily available without the need to hunt, trap or kill. However, our physiology is very similar to how it would've been in 10,000BC; evolution takes place at an incredibly slow pace. This means that our bodies largely respond to food in the *same way* our ancestors' bodies would've responded to food.

Our ancestors learned to identify the most valuable types of food (in terms of the valuable energy it contained) by the way it tasted. Anything that contained sugar was of great value; sugar provided energy to hunt and find more food. Anything that contained fat was also held in the highest regard. Fat provided warmth (while shielding their organs) and energy for many days. This is the reason why fatty and sugary foods taste *so* good to us now! It mostly comes down to evolution. We evolved to seek these foods and value them above other less energy-dense foods, simply because sweet fruit and fatty meat sustained the bodies of our ancestors.

Anyway, this puts us in quite a difficult position in the modern day. Sugary and fatty foods are all too readily available - you probably have some within your reach right now! So, while the availability of these once-coveted foods has changed, our physiology has not. We still crave these foods and your body still sees them as very valuable, which is why it can be so hard to say "no" to that slice of chocolate cake, even after a satisfying dinner.

The second problem is that, as a population, we are now the most sedentary we have ever been. We move only a fraction of the amount that our ancestors would have moved each day. We no longer need to hunt for our meals; we just hop in the car and drive to the shop. This means that many of us *burn* significantly fewer calories each day than we *consume*, making weight gain very easy. This also makes losing that weight, or staying at a healthy weight, very difficult.

Now, I know we're constantly told in the media and by our doctors, often brutally, that we need to lose weight. However, unless you know the reasoning behind why you should heed this advice, it's easy to pretend you haven't heard and carry on as you are. In this section of the book, I want to make a case for why a healthy weight is very important for your longevity and your quality of life. In the next section, we'll also talk about how to lose weight when exercise isn't an option.

So, why should we try to maintain a healthy weight throughout our lives? Being overweight carries significant risks. As well as putting you at risk of developing high blood pressure[44] and high cholesterol[45] (which constitutes a risky combination for heart disease), those who are overweight are also more likely to develop type-2 diabetes[46]. Certain types of cancer also occur more frequently in those who are overweight[47], and we see a higher incidence of stroke[48] in the same population.

Painful problems are also made worse, more often than not, by being overweight. Each extra pound you carry means an extra pound of weight traveling through any load-bearing joints, which is bad news for problems like arthritis and has been shown to lead to worse pain compared to those of a healthy weight[49]. People who are overweight tend to have worse blood chemistry as well, meaning their injuries recover slowly[50]. It is always more difficult to get people better when they're overweight compared to their fitter peers.

But that's enough doom and gloom about being overweight! Let's instead talk about the positives of being at a healthy weight:

- **Energy levels:** Being at a healthy weight will cause your energy levels to rise, helping you to feel ready to tackle whatever the day throws at you. Being overweight carries a high risk of lethargy and often leads to a big crash in the middle of the day.

- **Self-confidence:** Let's face it; no one enjoys being overweight. One of the reasons for this is the self-confidence issues carrying extra weight can cause. Maintaining a healthy weight leads to improved self-esteem (and often a better sex life as a result).

- **Ease of movement:** Those who were previously overweight and are now at a healthy weight often report to me how noticeable it is for them when they walk any significant distance or climb stairs. They remark about how easy it has become since shedding the pounds, and how little their knees now creak and ache during these activities. Do you have to lose all the excess weight to get these benefits? Nope! Most of my clients report noticeable changes after as little as five pounds of weight loss.

• **Improved stamina:** Similar to the point above, it can be embarrassing and frustrating to be out of breath at the top of a flight of stairs, or being unable to keep up with your partner when out walking. By losing unnecessary pounds, you'll have less weight on your body to carry when you walk, as well as improved heart and lung health. This means you can go on for longer before having to stop to catch your breath.

• **Less risk of injury:** People who are overweight tend to have a higher risk of elevated blood sugar levels[51]. Most people know about the link between high blood sugar and diabetes, but an uncontrolled blood sugar level also leads to harmful inflammation throughout the body. This can cause injury healing to slow down, as well as making the occurrence of certain "overuse" injuries more likely in the first place[50].

• **Living longer (and remaining independent and active):** A study[52] carried out by researchers from three Canadian Universities showed that obese men have a life expectancy *eight years* below the average, and may lose as many as *twenty* years of living in good health. Staying active and keeping a healthy weight means that there's every chance you'll get to spend more quality years with your loved ones.

So, now we've made a case for why maintaining a healthy weight is vital for over-fifties, let's discuss how you can get to that healthy weight… even when you're unable to exercise because of time constraints or a painful problem.

How to Lose Weight When You Can't Exercise

Many of my clients come to me with a frustrating conundrum: they have a painful condition, so they find it difficult to exercise because of the discomfort. As they can't exercise like they used to, they end up gaining weight against their will. As they're heavier with each day that goes past, the extra weight puts stress on their joints... making their painful problem worse. Can you see how this very easily becomes a vicious circle?

I'll be completely honest with you: losing weight when you can't exercise can be a very difficult thing to do. To make matters worse, your metabolism does indeed slow down as you go past fifty years of age, meaning you burn less calories each day doing the same things[53]. However, with discipline and persistence, it is possible to lose weight without exercise - you just need to know how.

When you can't take part in your regular form of exercise because it has become painful, it's important to experiment with other forms of exercise before writing it off entirely. For example, if you find it painful to walk, try swimming. If you can't swim, try riding your bike. If you have a gym membership, try the elliptical rather than the treadmill. Success will come down to trial and error, so be persistent and imaginative. To give you an example, when I had a client who suffered a broken ankle, she could no longer go to her Zumba class, which was her usual weekly exercise. Instead, we substituted the exercise from the class with a little dance routine she could do in a chair while holding some light dumbbells;

sounds easy, but after ten minutes, she was more than a little breathless. As soon as she was able to slightly weight bear on the ankle, we got her in the pool so she could walk up and down and swim, which turned out to be an excellent alternative.

If you really can't exercise after an injury, the only way you'll be able to lose weight is by making changes to your diet. This section is not for me to tell you what to eat and what not to eat; I'm simply going to explain the science behind food choices and weight loss, so you can make healthier decisions for your own circumstances.

The food we eat is largely composed of three "macronutrients", called protein, carbohydrate and fat.

Protein makes up the building blocks of muscle and is very important to a number of other bodily functions. Protein is found in meat, fish, eggs and nuts.

Carbohydrates provide an important energy source for us, found in bread, pasta, rice and potatoes.

And **fat** is arguably the most important of the macronutrients, allowing protection of our organs, hormonal balance and energy production.

Interestingly, you cannot survive without protein or fat for very long, but many people choose not to include carbohydrates in their diet and get along just fine[54].

Another important factor to consider is the way we measure the energy within our food. We call this unit of energy measurement a "calorie". You may have noticed the calories displayed on food packets. It is important to know a little about calories and what they mean to us when trying to lose weight.

Our bodies burn calories to survive. Each day, if we were to stay in bed all day and not move an inch, just by being alive we'd still burn a certain number of calories to keep our heart beating and our lungs breathing. That number goes up in direct proportion to how much movement and exercise we do each day, as well as due to a number of other factors.

If we all did exactly the same amount of exercise over the course of 24 hours, each of us would burn a different number of calories, which makes it difficult to make an assumption as to exactly how many calories you burn doing a given task. The national guidelines[55] state that men burn an average of 2500 calories each day, while women burn an average of 2000 calories each day. However, this figure can vary widely from person to person. One person may see weight gain from eating 2000 calories a day, where another may see significant weight loss from eating the same number of calories.

Ultimately, weight gain and weight loss simply comes down to how many calories you consume and how many calories your body burns[56]. If you consume more calories than you burn, you'll gain weight. If you consume less calories than you burn, you'll lose weight. However, this in isolation is too simplistic a view to take on diet. I could eat one McDonald's meal each day and nothing else and I would probably lose weight. However, I'd be far from healthy. Therefore, we need to go a little deeper and discuss how to lose weight in a healthy way.

Let's talk a little more about the macronutrients. The macronutrients make up the bulk of our meals, but each one has a different density of calories per gram. These calorific concentrations are as follows:

- **Protein**: 4 calories per gram

- **Carbohydrates**: 4 calories per gram
- **Fat**: 9 calories per gram

This is why fatty foods have historically been over-simplistically dubbed as "unhealthy" - because they contain more calories per unit of weight than carbohydrate-rich foods, for example. However, it is important to realise that there are no *good* or *bad* nutrients. They all have different jobs and are important to our bodies in different ways.

In order to lose weight, it's essential that we first know roughly how many calories it takes for us to sustain our current weight. Once we know this, if we want to gain weight, we add calories and if we want to lose weight, we subtract calories. The only straightforward way to tell how many calories it takes for you to maintain weight is to decide if you're currently gaining weight or staying the same based on your current diet. If you've been roughly the same weight for a few weeks, then great; you're probably at your current 'maintenance' level of calories. If you're gaining weight, you may need to cut out some calorific foods each day until you're able to maintain your weight for a week or two.

Once you know that what you're currently eating is giving you your maintenance level of calories, you could use a free food tracking app or website (I recommend MyFitnessPal: **https://www.myfitnesspal.com/**) to input your daily meals. The results from this programme will show you a detailed breakdown of how many calories you're consuming, as well as the ratio of fat, protein and carbohydrate in your diet.

In terms of ratios between these key nutrients, different ratios work best for different people. As a general rule for most people, it makes sense to keep protein reasonably high, then play around with fat and carbohydrates until you hit your 'target number' of calories each day. This may not be appropriate if you have a past history of kidney problems, so always get individual advice first. It's important to also include a wide variety of fruit and vegetables in your diet too as these contain "micronutrients" that keep us healthy.

You work out your target number of calories each day for weight loss by taking the number of calories that it takes to maintain your weight and subtracting between 100-500 calories from that, then using this new number as your goal each day. I would recommend going on to track the foods you eat in the MyFitnessPal app or website for at least a few weeks, so you get to grips with roughly how many calories are in each meal. I can tell you I was surprised when I did this for myself; some common foods in my diet had an incredibly high number of calories, while others filled me up but were low in calories.

While this approach does take discipline, it allows some margin for error; if you over-eat one day, you can make up for it on another day by eating slightly less - so the total evens out over the course of a week.

I've found this dieting approach to be the most consistently successful when followed. The regular "fad" diets that come out in the media never stick around for long as they tend to have major flaws; for example, the "weight loss tea" craze fell apart when it was shown that followers were getting severely dehydrated. The no-carbohydrate diet was great for rapid weight loss… but often led to rapid weight gain as soon as the person started eating carbohydrates again. Every day there is a new "proven", supposedly superior diet released by a "specialist", but going back to basics is consistently the best method.

If tracking your meals is too much effort for you, the general guidelines[57] for diet in the UK recommend that we eat plenty of fruit and vegetables, keep "trans fats" (processed foods) and sugar to a minimum, eat fatty foods in moderation, consume a diet rich in "slow-release" carbohydrates (like sweet potatoes and oats) and ensure we get a variety of proteins from eggs, meat and fish (or vegetarian sources if you don't eat animal products).

It's not up for debate whether weight is important when it comes to a painful problem; stress on the joints almost always leads to worse pain and the effects of being overweight on the body as a whole do tend to slow down healing. If you're struggling with your weight and truly cannot exercise, do go and speak to your doctor or a registered dietician to get some advice specific to your individual circumstances.

The last thing to say on this topic is to try not to get frustrated with yourself! Weight loss isn't easy and can be a frustrating process. It's quite common to see a few pounds of weight loss over the course of a few weeks, only for it to seem like you've put it all back on over one ill-disciplined weekend! But be persistent; just a small loss of weight can translate to significant improvements in health and injury, as well as safeguarding you from future problems. Work out a weight loss plan that works for you, and stick to it!

Coffee or Tea? Three Proven Benefits of Each

Are you a coffee or a tea person?

Coffee and tea have been a somewhat ritualistic tradition in our country over the last several hundred years. Tea was introduced to England in the 1660's by King Charles II and was predominantly a drink for the upper classes of society. However, by the eighteenth century, it was a drink for all social classes and tea consumption these days is estimated to be around 1.9kg per person, per year in the UK alone! Tea may have been discovered relatively late by us Brits; there are archives suggesting that the Chinese have been drinking tea since the third century BC.

Coffee was discovered by chance in Yemen, as the legend goes. A holy man was exiled from the kingdom of Mecca, and attempted to sustain his exhausted body by eating some berries from a plant during his wanderings. The berries tasted bitter, so he roasted them in an attempt to make them sweeter. However, the berries hardened after roasting, so the holy man tried to soften them by boiling them in water. The water turned into a fragrant, dark liquid and he decided to drink it. As the story goes, he was vitalised to such an extent that he was able to continue on his journey without needing to pause for rest or food for another *two* days!

Coffee was introduced to England in the same century as tea, according to reports. The first "coffee shop" in England was opened in Cornhill, London, and drinking coffee quickly became a ritual amongst middle-class citizens discussing politics and other worldly matters.

Fast forward four-hundred years, and not much has changed! We still use coffee to provide us with energy and we still drink tea with friends and family. Before we had the technology to investigate the health benefits of tea and coffee, our predecessors believed there were some medicinal effects associated with these drinks. And they just may have been right.

There are proven benefits of drinking both tea and coffee, and I've picked out three of the best to present to you here.

Benefits of Tea

- **Tea contains anti-oxidants:** Tea contains high levels of anti-oxidants: substances found in many foods that remove free radicals and limit cell damage within the body, protecting from nasties like heart disease and cancer[58]. Results of a recent study also showed that black tea had the potential to control blood sugar levels and stave off diabetes[59] - just don't undo that effect with two teaspoons of the sweet stuff!

- **Tea has been shown to have potential in the battle against high blood cholesterol.** A simplified view of cholesterol that many people take is that we should be trying to limit low-density lipoprotein (or "LDL") cholesterol in order to reduce the risk of certain heart diseases. In a study from 2008, researchers saw a 12% decrease in obese patients' LDL cholesterol just from 3 months of black tea consumption (without any of changes to their daily diet)[60].

- **Tea may reduce your risk of stroke.** One study chose almost 75,000 people to follow for over 10 years and correlated their black tea consumption with incidence of stroke. They found that those who drank four or more cups of tea each day had a 32% decrease in their risk of stroke[61]! While correlations don't necessarily point to cause and effect, medical professionals say that 80% of strokes are preventable by proper lifestyle choices, and this finding has been replicated in a similar study[62].

Benefits of Coffee

- **Coffee may protect against Alzheimer's:** There is strong evidence to suggest that the compounds in coffee (including caffeine) may help to break down the brain-plaques that cause Alzheimer's disease. Researchers found that drinking coffee led to a significantly reduced risk of the disease, independent of any other variables[63].

- **Coffee may protect against MS:** There is evidence to suggest that coffee drinkers have a reduced risk of developing multiple sclerosis. The researchers found that this was a dose-dependent effect, with those drinking more coffee less likely to suffer from the disease[64]. Again, this may be because of the documented neuro-protective effects of caffeine.

• **If you drink your coffee decaffeinated, don't fret!** There are studies showing the benefits of all types of coffee on a range of health problems. A 2016 study showed that those who drink one to two cups of coffee a day (regardless of type) had a 26% decreased risk of developing colorectal cancer[65]. This may be because of compounds called polyphenols contained in coffee, which work as anti-oxidants. Melanoidins, created in the coffee roasting process, may also help to improve colon mobility.

As a coffee-fanatic, I may be biased, but I saved the best benefit until last if you aren't yet convinced that coffee is your friend. In a study of over 3 million people funded by the National Cancer Institute, conducted over a twenty year period, people who drank 1-3 cups of coffee per day had an 18% decreased risk of death from ANY cause. Some of the diseases that were identified as having a decreased incidence in coffee drinkers included cancer, heart disease, respiratory disease, kidney disease and stroke[66]. Not bad for a little roasted berry drink, eh?

Watch Your Step(s)

No doubt you'll have heard about the magic 10,000-steps-per-day goal pushed by the media, community and even the government over the last few years. The question is, though, where did this 10,000 step goal come from and why are we encouraged to aim for it? I'd also like to pose a different question to you here: is there a quicker, easier way to get the same benefits, other than walking five miles every day?

It turns out that the 10,000 steps per day goal originated in Japan, in the 1960's. A Japanese University researcher became worried about the increasingly sedentary population in Japan. He hypothesised that asking people to raise their average steps from 3,500 per day to 10,000 per day would help them burn significantly more calories each week, combating weight gain and coronary heart disease. He created one of the earliest versions of a step-counter, which could be attached to the pocket and counted steps as it responded to vibrations.

The step counter was a success, along with the researcher's marketing strategy! Not only did Japan pick the ball up and run with it, other countries caught on too; and before long, 10,000 steps per day was seen as gospel. It turns out, since then, there hasn't actually been much further scientific research in support of this number.

Researchers have compared the health benefits of walking, say 3,500 steps against 10,000 steps, with the latter unsurprisingly being better for calorie burn and staving off heart disease; but there have been fewer studies comparing two higher step numbers, or whether a high step count is better than alternative exercise methods[67].

The average person in England walks between 3,500 and 5,000 steps per day[68]. Increasing that average to 10,000 would lead to an extra 500 calories burned per day, so 3,500 extra per week. This equates to roughly one pound of body fat lost (providing one's diet stays the same) - meaning, if diet is constant, increasing your steps from 3,500 to 10,000 each day should lead to roughly one pound of fat loss per week.

My concern around the 10,000 steps per day target, however, is that suddenly increasing your steps from a low count to a high count poses the risk of developing certain injuries. Rapidly changing your activity levels can lead to overuse injuries, like Achilles tendon problems or plantar fasciitis, which can firmly stop you in your tracks and make the whole exercise of trying to get fit pretty futile.

In a very small experiment covered by the BBC[69], professor Rob Copeland from Sheffield Hallam University wanted to investigate whether asking people to do three brisk 10-minute walks per day would be as beneficial to health as asking people to walk the full 10,000 steps (but at a leisurely pace) each day. The three walks represent about 1.5 miles of distance covered, as opposed to 5 miles with the 10,000 steps, and would represent significant time saved if it was as effective.

For this experiment, the participants in the three-walks group were asked to walk briskly and with purpose, rather than ambling along. When the results of the study came in, the three-walks group reported significantly less trouble sticking to the task than the 10,000 steps group. No surprises there. But when looking at the health benefits between the two groups, the three-walks group also came out on top. The researchers said that the brisk walking group checked off more "moderate exercise" minutes than the 10,000 steps group, even though the latter group spent far more time in total on their feet.

This is only a preliminary and very small study, but it gives us some important information about how it might be easier to stay fit and healthy than many media outlets (and even doctors) might have you believe. The key takeaway in this study, in my opinion, is how much more beneficial walking with intent is - to the point where you're out of breath - when compared to ambling along.

I know that many of my clients are shocked by how few steps they really do take each day when they start to count steps through a FitBit, app or smartwatch. When you feel as though you've been quite active but still aren't even halfway to the 10,000 step goal when you check at the end of the day, it can be demotivating and make it difficult to see how this goal is achievable for those of us with busy lives. By substituting your 10,000 step goal with three brisk 10-minute walks each day, the goalposts are suddenly shifted to a much more manageable place. Based on my own experience, and the results from studies like this, I've changed my recommendations to many clients; if you're not currently as active as you'd like, will you change your goal too?

Use the Sauna

Although I am biased in this suggestion as a regular sauna user myself, it looks as though the evidence is on my side on this occasion! I want to highlight to you some of the overwhelming evidence supporting sauna use in this section.

As an example, on study showed that the sauna has the potential to slash levels of norepinephrine (a stress hormone) in the blood[70]. This could be part of the mechanism behind the finding in a different study that three months use of the sauna improved self-reported stress, fatigue, and overall general health[71].

It isn't just wellbeing that improves with the sauna; six weeks of sauna use was shown to significantly decrease leg pain in those with arterial disease[72]. Sauna use also increases insulin-sensitivity[73]; meaning that your body can shuttle nutrients to muscles more efficiently, lowering blood sugar (which, if chronically elevated, can cause diabetes).

We can't forget to mention the mental health benefits; people who used the sauna over four times per week had a 66.7% decrease in their risk of Azheimer's Disease[74] and a 40% decrease in overall mortality over 20 years[75]. Just to clarify that last point: sauna use decreased the risk of death by *any* cause by a massive *40%* over a 20-year period! Use of the sauna even reduced the death rate of a group of very unwell cardiovascular patients by 6%[76].

Personally, I find that 15-minute sauna sessions profoundly help with my own wellbeing, recovery from exercise and the stresses of life. In addition to the points I've made so far, it has been shown that sauna sessions positively affect pain scores for a range of conditions[77,78] and I have found that using the sauna seems to dramatically speed up the time it takes me personally to recover from injury.

Luckily, the negative effects of the sauna seem to be minimal for most people[79]. You must be a bit careful with the light-headedness caused by the temporary drop in blood pressure, so always consult your doctor before starting a sauna regime.

Stressed, depressed or anxious individuals have the potential to see great improvements when adopting sauna use, too. Besides the physical benefits of sauna use, spending 15-minutes in a quiet room to sit with your own thoughts is a wonderful way to unwind, reflect and even meditate.

If possible, to get the greatest benefits from sauna use, I would recommend using the sauna at least three times per week if feasible and deemed appropriate by your doctor. In terms of duration, aim for 10-15 minutes each go. Give it four weeks and assess your stress, wellbeing and pain levels; if effective, it could be one of the most enjoyable ways to improve some of the problems that you may currently be facing!

Reaching for the Anti-Inflammatories? Consider Omega-3

While pain killers do undoubtedly help some people get relief from painful problems, they also come with a whole host of problems. For a start, opioid pain killers (like codeine and Oramorph) can be addictive. They also put stress on the liver during their transit through the body.

Some of the most prescribed medications for pain are in a family called *anti-inflammatory* pain killers. These include drugs like ibuprofen, Naproxen and Diclofenac. These drugs are known to cause potentially serious adverse effects, including stomach ulcers, gastric bleeding, heart attacks and even death. While they can be effective for pain, they should only be taken over the short-term. Prolonged use can lead to a whole host of health problems.

So, hopefully we can agree that reliance on prescription drugs for pain relief is usually a bad idea. But is there a safer alternative?

As a quick important note to you, I am not for one second suggesting that you stop taking any medication prescribed to you, or suggesting that you start any new supplement regime; I am merely reporting on findings in the evidence base, at the time of writing.

There is research to suggest that Omega-3 Fish Oils containing essential fatty acids may well be as, if not more, effective than traditional anti-inflammatory medication for back pain caused by disc bulges and degeneration, according to the journal Surgical Neurology[80]. This study showed that Omega-3 supplements have the potential to reduce the inflammatory response within the body, which may provide pain relief and improve recovery from some conditions.

The paper was published by two neurosurgeons who considered high doses of Omega-3 fish oil supplements as an alternative to traditional anti-inflammatories for their patients who complained of back or neck pain. The researchers recommended that the participants in their study consumed 1200mg of Omega-3 fish oil per day. As most Omega-3 supplements come in 300mg capsules, this is the equivalent of around 4 capsules, so quite a large dose. If you were to consider trying this at home, you'd definitely need to seek advice from your doctor beforehand.

The results were measured after an average of 75 days of supplementation and were very interesting:

- 59% of individuals had decided to stop taking their prescription pain medications because their symptoms had reduced so much.
- 60% stated that their overall pain had significantly improved.
- 80% of people in the study said that they were satisfied with the results they had seen.
- 88% of people in the study said that they would continue to take the Omega-3 fish oil supplement.
- Perhaps most importantly – no subjects reported any adverse effects as a result of the Omega-3 supplement.

When you compare the results of this study to those of the usual pain killer trials, there are usually multiple adverse effects reported and less of a positive effect observed.

In my humble opinion, I think it is worth seriously considering Omega-3 as one of the most important supplements for many people, not just those with a painful problem. The reason for this is partly because of the positive effects Omega-3 can bring to general health - and partly because most of us chronically fail to consume enough Omega-3 as part of our normal diets.

However, before you reach for the supplements, there are some important points to consider. For a start, not all Omega-3 supplements are created equal. Some are of far superior quality when compared to others, and quality matters greatly. It may even be *harmful* to take poor quality omega-3 supplements over a prolonged period of time due to the vitamin A and possible mercury content. Some experts say that poor quality Omega-3 supplements with a "fishy" smell may genuinely have a high level of rancidity, too[81]; not a pleasant thought. I should also mention that it is almost always best to get as much of any particular vitamin or nutrient through whole food sources as opposed to supplements wherever you possibly can.

Here are some great ways to add more natural Omega-3 into your diet:

- **Oily fish** – not surprisingly, oily fish contain a high concentration of Omega-3. Fish like salmon, mackerel and sardines are full of Omega-3, but you can still find a smaller amount in white fish too.

- **Nuts** – walnuts, cashew nuts and almonds all contain high levels of Omega-3.

- **Green leafy vegetables** – packed with vitamins and minerals, including Omega-3, green leafy veg is an essential part of any diet.

- **Omega-3 supplements** - for most people, an Omega-3 supplement is an easy and convenient way to include more of this powerful super-nutrient in your diet. The British Dietician's Association[82] recommends looking for supplements that explicitly state "Omega-3" rather than "Cod Liver Oil". They also recommend that the general population limits their Vitamin A content to below 1500ug/day and also seeks out a high quality supplement. Check the label of your supplements and consult a dietician for advice on how to maintain this guideline. My general advice would be that you usually get what you pay for - the £1 supermarket Omega-3 supplements are often of very poor quality, so do your research before parting with your money.

Whole Body Cooling

We've already talked about the power of heating your body through use of a sauna, but did you know that harnessing the power of cold can have an even greater effect on pain for many people?

It has long been accepted that extremely cold temperatures (-67°C) are effective for reducing inflammation[83], dampening the experience of pain[84] and even encouraging weight loss[85]. They are also very effective for enhancing range of motion and decreasing muscle spasm in people with lower back pain. One study[86] found that out of two groups of men with back pain who completed an exercise programme, the group that was first given whole body cooling had less lower back muscle spasm and a far greater range of spinal motion than the other group.

So, how does this effect from cooling occur?

There are physical *and* hormonal effects on the human body that come about because of cold exposure. These can be so powerful that people have dedicated their whole lives to researching the healing effects of cold on the human body. Some even say that the reason Scandinavian people tend to be healthier than most other groups is partly because of the regular cold exposure in their lifestyle; ice-cold plunge pools are a way of life for some Scandinavian communities.

Am I saying you need to remove the peas and frozen chicken from your freezer and climb in there yourself? Not necessarily.

A 2015 study published in the *European Journal of Physical Rehabilitative Medicine* showed that we might be able to achieve the same positive effects for people with pain in less extreme temperatures[87]. The researchers in this study took a group of people with chronic low back pain and placed them in one of two cold chambers – one was -67°C and one was -5°C. Their results demonstrated significant pain relief in both conditions, but neither condition was superior to the other.

There are some effective ways of cooling the entire body for pain relief, with a view to repeating the results of that study. One such method involves exposing yourself to the cold with a quick five-minute cold blast at the end of a shower. It is important to mention that cold exposure is not suitable for everyone and some people find the cold can *worsen* muscle spasm rather than improve it. Be sure to check with your doctor before attempting the following exercises.

This method sounds easy, but usually requires some build-up over a few weeks. To start with, try to endure 10-second cold blasts at the end of every shower just before you get out for one week. Build these quick blasts up to at least 30-seconds before you try the technique below.

Take a shower at your usual temperature, for your usual duration of time. Before you get out, turn the hot water off and turn the cold water on full. Stand facing the water for 2-minutes so that it is hitting your chest. Next, drop your head forward so that the water is running off the top of your head. Finally, turn away from the shower, so that the cold water is first hitting your neck, then running down your back. Stand in this position for a further 2-minutes.

I have tested the optimal length of time that I felt it took to get positive effects with cold showers myself. You can certainly feel invigorated, energised and less achy after a 30-second cold blast, but the real benefits start at 5-minute efforts.

This powerful technique might feel like a real challenge at first but when you get into the habit of enduring the quick blast each day, it becomes exhilarating. I got to a stage within about two weeks where I would look forward to the cold shock (I opted for mine post-workout). This method may suit people suffering from any kind of inflammation-related pain. It significantly helped my shoulder when I was suffering from a tear in the cartilage around the joint.

Although there is some evidence to suggest the cold can help muscle pain, if your pain is caused by muscle spasms you might want to skip this technique until they settle down. This is because a cold "shock" can sometimes cause the muscles to tense up further. People with muscle spasm might want to opt for heat treatment instead. As always, check with your doctor who will be able to tell you which method is most suitable for your personal circumstances.

Eat This, Not That

Did you know that the food you eat plays a major role not just in your weight but also in how quickly you recover from injury? There are foods that encourage rapid healing; reducing inflammation and promoting general wellbeing. There are other foods that produce a cascade of negative effects; elevating blood sugar, grinding healing to a halt and causing inflammatory chemicals to swirl in our blood stream.

In this instance, knowledge is power. If you know which foods to avoid, you can replace them with the foods that will produce the opposite effect. Remember, each meal you eat provides a unique opportunity to take a step *towards* being pain-free, rather than away from it.

Some of the foods in the following list of recommended substitutions are already widely recognised as being healthy, while others may surprise you. *Please note:* as always, I can't tell you what or what not to eat. You must make this decision for yourself following a consultation with your doctor or dietician. That being said, here are some general tips which you may find helpful:

- Instead of fizzy drinks containing sugar or huge amounts of aspartame (a sweetener considered harmful by many), choose **iced water with the juice of half a lime** squeezed in. I start every day with this brilliantly simple drink in place of my morning coffee. In order to fully recover from injury, we should ditch the fizzy drinks as sugar and aspartame have been shown to raise levels of inflammatory chemicals in the human body[88].

- Instead of vegetable or sunflower oil, choose **coconut or extra virgin olive oil**. Vegetable oil (which is also found in mayonnaise and BBQ sauce) contains compounds which raise levels of inflammatory hormones as well as encouraging the body to store fat. Coconut oil, on the other hand, has inherent anti-oxidant properties and some experts suggest its daily use can help to stave off illnesses caused by oxidisation, including cancer[89]. In this way, it can actually be used to *help* weight loss, counter-intuitively. Extra virgin olive oil has anti-inflammatory properties when used in moderate quantities and in my opinion makes food taste far better than vegetable oil.

- Instead of fried, processed crisps, try your own **homemade vegetable chips**. As well as the fact that fried, processed foods have usually been cooked in vegetable oil, they can lead to weight gain when consumed often - with excess weight often causing pressure on joints and worsening painful problems. As a substitute, try **homemade kale crisps**. They taste much better than they sound and involve minimal preparation. Place foil over a baking tray, then cover it with kale. Lightly drizzle the kale with extra virgin olive oil and salt and pepper. Place the tray into an oven on 180°C and bake for 25-minutes. The kale crisps should be crunchy and packed with flavour, making an excellent potato crisp substitute, packed with anti-inflammatory properties.

- Instead of wheat and gluten products, try **gluten-free alternatives or sweet potato**. Gluten-based foods like bread and pasta have been linked with a whole slew of health detriments[90]. Some experts even believe that we are all gluten-intolerant (coeliac) to a certain degree. Gluten-based foods can wreak havoc on the gastric tract, causing bloating, discomfort and lethargy. Why not replace your usual gluten-based foods with either the store-bought gluten-free version, or a creative alternative, using ingredients like cauliflower and sweet potato? Search for "cauliflower pizza base" online or "sweet potato burger buns" for some great gluten replacement ideas.

Other Dietary Additions to Consider

- **Tomatoes** are packed with anti-oxidants, vitamins and minerals which will all support the body throughout the natural healing process.

- In addition to kale that we mentioned earlier, **broccoli, collard greens** and **sprouts** all hold similar anti-oxidising properties, along with vitamins A, C and K. They help to stabilise blood sugar levels by regulating spikes in insulin.

- **Almonds, cashews** and **Brazil nuts** all contain high levels of Omega-3, a well-established anti-inflammatory. These nuts also contain "*phytonutrients*" which promote healing and will keep you fuller for longer when used as a mid-morning snack.

- **Bok Choi**, common in Chinese dishes, boasts an impressive *seventy* different anti-oxidising minerals!

- **Blueberries** contain quercetin, a natural substance that can ward off inflammation. These little berries have long been established as a "superfood".

- **Pineapple** contains a digestive enzyme that helps to break down inflammatory cells. Do remember to only consume pineapple in small to moderate quantities, due to its high fructose content (more on that in the next chapter).

Avoid Fruit Juice

While the saying has always been *"an apple a day keeps the doctor away"*, there may be a caveat to this. I fully accept that eating fruit has health benefits; oranges *can* improve your immunity[91] and apples *do* contain important vitamins. However, eating fruit is a far cry away from drinking fruit juices, even when they are labelled 100% pure.

While all fruits contains fructose, this simple sugar is found in only moderate quantities in whole fruit. Despite the scare-mongering that you might read online, eating 3-5 pieces of fruit per day is **not** likely to be enough to cause fructose-related problems; which include the risk of developing diabetes, increasing levels of inflammation and frequent energy crashes.

However, fruit *juice*, particularly from concentrate, *does* contain high levels of this simple sugar that can have unwanted effects inside the body.

Substituting fruit juice for water is the ideal swap. However, a lot of people find drinking water unpleasant, so adding a cordial or squash with minimal sugar or added sweetener can help to satisfy the cravings for sweetness.

Anyone trying to lose weight should put this substitute into action without delay. People not worried about their weight or blood sugar but who have a painful problem can also benefit. If you are suffering from a tendon problem, there is some evidence to suggest that cutting back on sugars (like fructose) should be a priority too[92].

CHAPTER EIGHT

Well-Being & The Power of Your Mind

Introduction

Once upon a time, society - and the medical profession alike - believed that pain could always be attributed to physical damage. If you had pain, it was because there was a physical, tangible, measurable problem. We also believed that just as the problem appeared in the first place, the moment it resolved, pain would disappear without a trace.

However, there was a problem with this theory. The advent of modern imaging technology revealed that it is entirely possible for someone to feel pain, with a complete *absence* of physical injury.

In the modern day, our medical imaging technology has improved vastly beyond the basic X-rays we've been able to perform for the last hundred years. We can now pick up on more physical problems in someone's body than ever before with the advent of the MRI scan. This has led to the use of MRI scans as the preferred diagnostic tool for many painful problems.

We initially thought that, surely, in everyone with a painful complaint, we would be able to see exactly what was causing the problem with our clever scans, knowing then what we needed to do to fix it.

Except, to the befuddlement of the medical profession, there were daily exceptions to this rule. People were in pain – in the absence of any discernible injury on their MRI scan. To make matters more confusing still, other people had no pain – yet we found degenerative discs, joint arthritis and even vertebral fractures seen on *their* scans!

An important study by Brinjikji and colleagues carried out in 2014 looked at the spines of a population of healthy individuals who were not complaining about any kind of back pain[1].

The researchers took these people and performed a full spinal MRI on each. The results were astonishing.

The researchers found that, out of **3,110** people:

- Up to 96% of these (pain-free) subjects had disc degeneration.
- There were disc bulges in 30% of the 20-year olds, and 84% of the 80-year olds.
- The was a disc protruding from the spine in up to 43% of these pain-free people.
- There was some evidence of "wear and tear" in nearly everyone.

And yet, despite all the focus in pain science being placed firmly on *physical* problems for hundreds of years, these people with seemingly horrific imaging results stood before us – without any pain whatsoever.

What's more, this study is not alone – it has been replicated time and time again, including areas of the body other than the spine[2,3].

So, how do we explain how some people experience terrible pain when they are in the exact same physical state as someone who is pain-free? There is clearly more at play than just the physical.

The human mind is a fantastic creation. It allows us to think, feel and understand. It can also amplify or suppress pain signals based upon our past experiences, current mood, subconscious fears and vulnerabilities[4]. This chapter is all about learning how to harness the power of the *mind* to control your pain. If you can use your mind to your advantage, it can work with you as a powerful ally, helping you control your pain - as opposed to having it blow out of all proportion.

Some of my biggest client success stories started off with a skeptical individual resisting this approach. Too many times to count, these individuals end up finding themselves die-hard believers in the power of the mind by the end of our time together.

Each one of the following tips has been carefully considered. I have distilled these tips down to the ones I feel are most effective. I would recommend trying them all for at least one week (unless otherwise stated) before making a judgment. Of course, some will take longer to work than others. Some may give you an instant boost, while others will take practice and patience. Some will not be suitable for your circumstances, so as with everything in this book, seek professional advice first if you're not sure. Without delaying any longer, here are my tips for using the magnificent capabilities of your mind to help you unlock your body and ease your pain.

Your New Mantra

Out of all the emotions that a human being can possibly experience in the context of pain, one of the most harmful, without doubt, is **fear.**

Fear, in the context of pain, causes us to avoid movements and activities that are safe and necessary for a complete recovery. One of the strongest types of fear is the fear of getting physically hurt. The fear of damaging our bodies. The fear of causing considerable pain.

This type of fear lies beneath the surface — we aren't necessarily aware of it — which limits your grip on the fear, even when you are determined to control it. Even if you don't *feel* afraid, your brain may be subconsciously fearful of the actions that have previously caused you pain; whether that be bending forward to pick something up off the floor, using the hoover or walking to the shops.

Our brains are programmed to learn. We learn through experiences, with any experience that has caused us significant pain (or enjoyment) being the most influential teachers. Your brain is very clever; it is entirely reasonable to develop fear towards a movement that caused you pain in the first place. After all, your brain is designed primarily to protect you from danger. Developing fear, and consequently avoidance, of a situation that the brain interprets as 'dangerous' is a mechanism that is designed to protect you.

However, there is one thing that our brains are programmed to believe that isn't necessarily true. Your brain believes that anything that causes you pain is *physically damaging* to your body. Lorimer Moseley (an

Australian world-renowned back pain expert) explained this phenomenon using one of his personal experiences[5].

He recounted walking through the long grasses near his home, when he felt what he assumed to be a fallen twig jab him in the calf.

Thinking nothing of it, he continued his walk.

As it turned out, the "twig" that had jabbed him was a deadly brown snake sinking its fangs into his lower leg. Lorimer ended up in hospital, fighting for his life, in desperate need of an anti-venom.

Luckily, he lived to tell the tale. The next time he went walking in a grassy field, he genuinely did get jabbed by a twig disguised in the long grass. What do you think he felt in his leg this time? If you said incredible, searing pain, you would be correct.

Why was his reaction this time so different to the innocuous snake bite months earlier? It was because of *learned fear*, etched into his mind by such a significant experience as almost losing his life.

Your brain is no different. If you've injured your body, your mind is on high alert, looking to avoid anything that represents a threat. At the first sign of this threat, your body is going to protect you in the only way it knows how – by producing pain, which tells you to STOP!

How do you stop this reaction and ease the unnecessary pain caused by your brain trying to protect you? It takes work, but I've found a simple mantra that can alleviate this reaction when repeated silently in your head.

This mantra is designed to work on movements that you could once do without pain — but have now become difficult. For example, someone with back pain who now fears bending forward to put their socks on.

The mantra is this:

"This pain does not mean I am damaging my body."

Next time you feel yourself aching at the mere thought of carrying out an activity that was once painful, remind yourself that pain does not equal damage. For it to work, you need to truly believe it. Luckily, research has shown that just repeating a certain phrase can solidify our belief in it, so keep reinforcing it with regular repetition if you can[6].

I've found this tip to be super-effective for people with conditions like fibromyalgia, if used over the long-term. Fibromyalgia can cause unexplained pain, seemingly with no rhyme or reason behind what hurts and what doesn't. Reminding yourself that your pain doesn't mean you are causing yourself physical harm should help to ease the anxiety associated with ongoing pain, as well as potentially the pain itself.

It takes practice, but the rewards are worth it.

Learn to Meditate

What do you think of when you hear the word "meditation"? Do you think of Buddhist monks sat cross-legged on a hard, stone floor for days on end chanting *"Ohm"*?

Fortunately, meditation for us average folk doesn't need to be such a feat of endurance, nor does it need to be spiritual if you don't want it to be. Meditation is the act of taking a short period of time to focus *inwardly* on yourself. And no, you do not need to be the *"enlightened one"* to gain some benefit from this practice! Meditation is a very simple process and the best part is: you can't meditate "wrong", because there is no "wrong"!

There are many types of meditation available to choose from, but most types focus around concentrating solely on noticing your breath entering and leaving your body. Most people prefer to sit still in a quiet place while they do this, but there's no reason why you can't focus on your breathing whilst going about your daily errands. When done consistently every day over ten days or so, for 20-minutes each day, I've found there to be a tangible sense of relaxation as a reward, extending long beyond the meditation time itself.

Meditation has been used to manage pain for hundreds of years by Buddhists. The effects of meditation on pain management have been, at last, tested in the West. In a 2018 review, the authors found that mindfulness meditation reduced self-reported pain significantly in chronic pain sufferers[7].

The authors of the aforementioned study attributed this to a change in the way the participants were "processing" their pain, thus reducing the unpleasant experience. No matter which way meditation works, the cost of implementing meditation into your daily routine is minimal. All it takes is 20-minutes of your time and a quiet space.

Most people opt to undertake their meditation practice first thing after they wake up, as their mind is clearer before the hubbub of every day life. When I say "first thing" is best, I really do mean first thing – this includes delaying your morning ritual of checking phones, the newspaper, emails or falling into "fire-fighting mode": the state of frantically trying to solve any problems or chores you may have that day as quickly as you can!

I believe that meditation must be performed every day for a minimum of ten days before you start to really feel the positive effects. Don't worry if you find it hard to concentrate on keeping your mind calm for twenty minutes. Some meditation masters suggest that achieving even *one* truly focussed breath per day is a good start!

Try this meditation practice below for ten days before evaluating the effects:

Find a quiet place to sit. You can choose any position, but I prefer to be upright (as I'll be less likely to fall asleep!) Close your eyes and focus on taking three deep breaths. Notice how the air enters and exits through your nose, how it rushes into your chest. Notice the area of your body that rises and falls as you breathe.

After these three initial breaths, with each new breath focus on a different part of the body. Simply observe how this part of the body feels as you breathe in and as you breathe out. Be very specific. For example, don't just focus on your hand. Focus on the second knuckle of your third finger. Change your focus each breath.

This tip is perfect for those suffering from chronic, low-level anxiety, which has been shown to significantly exacerbate painful problems. Classically, type-A personalities (high achievers who can't switch off) are the worst affected by this type of anxiety. We know that anxiety can worsen physical pain, so by putting measures in place to control it we can have a direct effect on physical pain too.

What's more, meditation has profound effects on productivity – taking the time to get your thoughts in order first thing in the morning can set your day up to be an ordered success rather than a chaotic scramble.

There is also some solid evidence behind the positive effects of mindfulness meditation on chronic headaches – researchers at the Baqiyatallah Hospital and Headache Clinic in 2018 found that mindfulness improved levels of disability, quality of life and reduced distress in chronic headache sufferers[8].

How Stress Could Be Ageing You Faster

We all deal with stress every single day. It's a part of life and sometimes stress can even be a good thing; certain types of stress spur us on to take action. If you've ever found an overdue bill (threatening a hefty fine) under a stack of papers you'll have experienced this sudden rush of stress-induced urgency. However, chronic, low-level (or indeed overwhelming) stress can be harmful in the long run, both to physical and mental health.

When we think of stress, we think about someone on the verge of a mental breakdown, at risk of "snapping" at any moment. While we all experience occasional times like this, they usually pass within a day or so. Beneath-the-surface, low-level, continuous stress, however, is a different ball game. This type of stress often goes undetected for long periods of time. It can be driven by a family problem, like watching the sad decline of an ageing family member, or at work, such as when we are put under sustained pressure with a looming deadline.

I like to think of this type of stress as water simmering in a pot on the stove. Slowly, the heat builds and you start to see bubbles, which at first burst harmlessly when they reach the surface as the water boils. However, if left unchecked, the boiling water can bubble up uncontrollably and even dislodge the lid covering the saucepan. When stress reaches boiling point, it's already too late - and similar to the example above, there's often a mess to clean up afterwards!

Low-level, unremitting stress can have a number of effects on our health, some of which we don't necessarily notice, or even associate with stress[9]. Stomach not feeling quite right? That's often stress-related. Did you think those headaches were down to not drinking enough water? Again, it could be stress simmering away. Have you lost your energy or sex drive? It could just be that you're getting to bed too late... but if there's a lot going on right now, you might need to look inwards instead.

Stress causes a lot of these effects on your body by releasing a hormone into your bloodstream called *cortisol*. Cortisol is a '*fight or flight*' hormone - meaning it is designed to force you to take action. In 50,000BC, when our ancestors were chased by prehistoric dinosaurs, cortisol made sure they could get away quickly. Unfortunately, our physiology hasn't changed very much since then; so, when someone shouts at you at work, your brain sends a signal to the adrenal glands to release into your bloodstream a similar dose of cortisol to the one your ancestors would've received when chased by that dinosaur. After all, your brain has perceived a threat in exactly the same way as it would've done 50,000 years ago. While you don't necessarily feel like getting up and running away, the effect on your body is the same.

Over time, this repeated dumping of cortisol into the bloodstream, day after day, month after month, can lead to permanent health problems[10]. Cortisol causes the body to switch off non-urgent systems, such as your immune and digestive systems, in favour of supplying energy to your heart and muscles. Great when we are running from danger - but not good when occurring repeatedly over long periods of time. Chronically elevated cortisol causes your immunity to take a dip and leaves you vulnerable to infection, as well as possibly even cancer, some experts say[11]. We're also less able to extract the nutrients we need from food as our digestive systems aren't fully functional in this state. Chronic, long-term stress has also been linked to anxiety, depression, heart disease, weight gain and memory impairment[12].

So, what can we do to "switch off" this ancient mechanism embedded deep in our brains, so we can get some relief from low-level, continuous fight-or-flight responses?

Experts say the following can help:

- Eating well, staying hydrated and regular exercise can all help[13]. Some highly successful people advocate the approach of making changes to the *body* first, which then encourages the brain to follow. If you've ever felt low, then gone for a brisk walk or run and not felt so bad after, you'll have experienced this at work.

- Learning to relax with Yoga, Tai Chi, or meditation has been shown to significantly relieve stress in a wide ranging population over a number of studies[14]. Most towns have plenty of choice when it comes to classes like these and I advise many clients to look into finding one to suit their needs. The best part is, the techniques you learn from these classes can be used outside of the class whenever you need a boost.

- Scheduling in time for your favourite hobbies, or even just to read a book, is important for managing stress. The key word in the previous sentence is *scheduling*. These activities need to be planned in advance, or they simply won't get done. When I started writing this book, I decided I was going to try and write a page or so whenever I "got a moment" to do so. Guess what? It never happened. So, I started scheduling in one hour every morning before work to sit down and write. I found the process relaxing and rewarding (and ended up completing the book on schedule too).

• Fostering and keeping healthy relationships may be the most important factor in controlling stress. Research has consistently demonstrated anxiety and depression rates to be higher in lonely individuals[15]. Sharing our worries with trusted companions is important and allows us to lift the lid from our "stress saucepans", even just for a moment. But it needn't all be doom and gloom that we share in order to benefit from a friend's company. Good times are equally important and allow you to switch off from the problems you might be going through in your life right now.

• Laughing and stoking the fire on your sense of humour is vital. Watch a comedy, or go and meet a friend who can always make you laugh. It's a great release valve for chronic stress when you put the world to rights with a healthy dose of humour.

• If you feel weighed down by the stress and strain of life and can't see a way out, seek help. There are trained professionals who specialise in helping people with problems just like this. They can help you find a way through. If you're in need of someone to talk to, your local GP surgery should have information about free services in your area. If you have the means to pay, I've never met anyone who has been through the process of therapy and described it as a waste of money. A skilled therapist can help you work through issues that you may not even realise are affecting you.

Use the Incredible Power of Touch

When you've suffered from pain for longer than twelve weeks, there are certain physical changes that occur in your brain and nervous system[16]. These changes can be the reason why some people find their physical injury has healed, yet their pain continues.

The changes I am talking about are characterised by heightened sensitivity in the nerves, both around the problem area and in the spinal cord leading up to the brain. This sensitivity can cause very real pain even in the total absence of damage.

Unfortunately, this can cause people to spiral into a vicious circle:

- You start to feel pain, often from an initially innocuous injury.
- This pain causes your nervous system to become *hyper-sensitive*, so the pain gets worse.
- This increase in pain causes your nervous system to become more sensitive still, leading to even more pain.
- The cycle repeats, ad nauseum. Not a good pattern.

These cycles are extremely hard to break. However, one of the most powerful tools we have in our arsenal is the power of *touch* from a loved one. Amazingly, when loved ones spend time together, their heartbeats and breathing patterns tend to naturally synchronise[17].

However, the effect of being with someone close to us doesn't end there. Touch can truly be a healing power. In a 2017 study, Dr Pavel Goldstein, a postdoctoral pain researcher in the Cognitive and Affective Neuroscience Lab at Colorado University, compared a woman's painful experiences both with and without her partner's touch[17]. Dr Goldstein found that the touch of her partner significantly reduced the magnitude of the woman's painful experience, more so than him just being present with her but not holding hands.

What caused such a profound change? The researchers felt that the level of trust between the couple played a significant role. The woman experiencing the pain had enough trust in her partner to believe that he was *physically sharing* the pain with her – and we all know that a problem shared is a problem halved.

By having someone we truly trust **lightly touch** a painful area with no more than the weight of a feather, the nerve signals this produces can help to calm the nervous system, reducing pain as a result. Asking a loved one to perform this simple act for you while relaxing in front of the television can make a world of difference to your symptoms.

Their touch is effectively telling your nervous system: *"Be calm, everything is OK. Look, this touch is safe and comfortable. You don't need to be on edge."*

INTO PRACTICE

Lie still on your side or back, either with some relaxing music on or in front of some light-hearted television.

Have your partner or trusted friend sit behind you, lightly brushing your back with their fingertips, moving slowly across your skin.

If it feels like a massage, they are pressing too hard!

Ask them to perform this for up to 30-minutes. You should feel a deep sense of relaxation which grows as time goes on. Do this daily for a week and re-evaluate your pain at the end of the week.

This technique requires patience but is primarily aimed at those suffering from what we call *"central sensitisation"* – that is, a painful response that may be caused by neuro-inflammation, or the response of the nervous system, rather than the injury itself[18]. If you've had scans and other investigations and they've come back showing no significant damage yet you still feel considerable pain, this may be for you. I have had clients with chronic back pain observe significant benefits from this technique in several weeks of practice.

Re-Invigorate Your Sex Life!

Did you know that people who have suffered from a painful problem for over twelve weeks are more likely to report a lack of sexual desire and satisfaction[19]?

To me, that isn't surprising. Being in pain is clearly not a turn-on for the sufferer. However, what did originally surprise me is learning that sex (more specifically, the chemicals released into our bloodstreams during intercourse) can have a dramatic and positive effect on pain[20].

When you think about what happens during sex, it really isn't all that surprising; the endorphins (feel-good chemicals) released during sex interact with the opiate receptors in our brains in a similar way to drugs such as codeine or morphine. So, it appears there *is* a way to get similar positive pain-relieving benefits of these pain killers without suffering any of the nasty side effects.

There doesn't appear to be any research on a minimum frequency required to experience the positive effects of sex on pain, but as the pain-killing effects seem to be transient, I would suggest that more is better!

In terms of practicality, I know that when you're struggling with easily-irritable pain, sex can be a logistical challenge. That's why I've done the research (just reading, I promise) to find out which positions might be the most comfortable, depending on what aggravates or eases your pain.

I have chosen to focus on the two problems that have the most negative impact on the sex lives of the clients I treat – hip pain and back pain.

For Women with Back Pain

If your pain gets worse when you bend forward, you might want to try a variation of the *"cowgirl"* position – where you sit astride your partner, knees supported on the bed.

Instead of sitting upright in this position, you'll want to lean back and support your body weight by placing your hands on your partners shins.

This position was shown to be one of the most comfortable for women who don't like to bend forwards by researchers in the European Spine Journal in 2015[21].

Alternatively, if you're fine bending forwards but standing, walking and leaning back triggers your back pain, you might want to try a variation of the traditional "missionary" position, say the same researchers.

You can either go for the classic missionary position (you laid on your back with knees bent, man on top), or a raunchier progression (your legs up, knees against his chest, man on top).

For Men with Back Pain

Gents, if your pain is worse when you bend forward, you will find most ease in a modified "cowgirl" position. This will involve your partner going on top, leaning forward, while you lay completely flat below her. This was the top recommended position for men who have difficulty flexing forward by Stuart McGill, world-renowned back pain researcher[22].

If you are fine bending forwards but have difficulty walking, standing or leaning back because of back pain, you may have most luck in a side-lying position.

For this position, your partner should lay on her side, facing away from you, with her knees and hips bent up slightly. You will lay on your side pressed up against her back, with a similar body shape to her. This position will limit any "extension" movement from the lower back and should feel the most comfortable.

For Women with Hip Pain

With hip pain caused by arthritis or other ageing changes, the hips lose significant mobility. Unfortunately, this can occur rapidly. For this reason, we need to use a position that avoids the commonly restricted hip movements.

The main three limited movements tend to be:

1. **Internal rotation** (turning the top of your thigh inwards to "face" the other thigh)

2. **Abduction** (spreading your legs apart)

3. **Flexion** (bringing your knee up to your chest)

If we think technically about the sex positions that involve these movements, quite a few of the traditional positions might be ruled out.

Missionary position involves the woman abducting her legs. Cowgirl (woman on top) involves internal rotation to allow the legs to straddle either side of her partner.

There is, however, an effective position that limits all three of these actions while remaining comfortable for both parties. It is a type of modified all-fours position and this is the position that was reported to be most comfortable for the people with hip pain that I surveyed during my research for this book.

It involves the woman lying face down, upper half supported by the bed, with her knees supported on the floor. If she shuffles her body forward, she can increase the angle between her thigh and her body to ease away from hip flexion, if this is an uncomfortable action. The man is then able to enter her from behind, without the need for her to spread her legs into abduction.

For Men with Hip Pain

In traditional missionary, it is the thrusting of the man that provides the motion during sex. With hip pain, this thrusting action can be real agony for the man and lead to a poor experience all round, with considerable pain afterwards.

If you are a male with hip pain and limited range of motion, the woman may have to start taking the lead in "female-dominant" positions. The cowgirl and reverse cowgirl (woman facing away) are great options in this case, as described in the sections above.

Harness the Power of Swearing!

An interesting 2009 paper in the journal *Neuroreport* showed that swearing while experiencing pain has the power to increase pain thresholds, increase heart rate and decrease perceived pain[23].

The subjects in this study were either asked to swear or say a non-swear word as they were poked and prodded. The results showed that the people in the swearing condition coped better with the pain and were able to continue further in the experiment before calling it quits.

But not so fast, potty mouth! The same researchers got back at it in 2011 to test whether this effect was as apparent in habitual swearers as it was in people who rarely swear. He found that those of us who swear like sailors are less likely to experience the positive effects of a quick cuss following a painful jolt or spasm than the more eloquently-spoken[24].

The researchers thought that this effect became apparent because swearing is linked to a quick emotional flare; however, we can become anaesthetised to this effect if we are using bad language multiple times every sentence.

The remedy to this is simple; try to save your naughty words for painful days and take on the vocabulary of your local vicar when you're having a more comfortable time.

Journaling to Track Progress

The premise behind this tip lies in the fact that if you can measure it, you can change it.

When we are afflicted by a painful condition, it is easy for the days to merge into one great, big, dark cloud. However, this experience prevents us from picking up on patterns and themes that might otherwise be useful.

You might find that one day brings only a fraction of the pain suffered on the other days of that week. However, if you haven't made a note of what you did to affect that change in the first place, you have no hope of repeating it.

Journaling has the potential to help us improve across many aspects of our lives. Journaling can help us measure the results of our business ventures, track our health and fitness, hit goals more efficiently, and organise our thoughts from an illogical mess into intelligible harmony.

I would recommend taking five minutes at the end of each day to track the following:

- Time you woke up
- How you slept and how you felt when you woke up (on a 1-10 scale if this makes it easier)
- Brief description of the foods you ate for each meal
- How your pain was in the morning, afternoon and evening
- Anything that made your pain better and anything that made it worse

Through the simple act of recording these things, you can actually improve them *without even trying*.

This is because of something called the *Hawthorne Effect* – we are more likely to make better decisions when we know we are being observed, or when we are accountable to something, even if it is just writing it down at the end of the day[25].

I've found that when I am tracking what I eat, for example, I make better choices. Why? It's not because I would rather eat healthy meals that day – it's because I know I have to write down whatever I put in my mouth (and the embarrassment of writing down "12 Maryland cookies" that evening is not something I wish to experience more than once).

This method is especially good for anyone who is a little overweight and struggles to shift the pounds. Being overweight can cause significantly greater discomfort to people with back pain, knee pain and hip pain. The sheer act of writing down what we eat each day helps to influence our choices and allows us to see where we might be going wrong.

Journaling is also great for anyone with chronic pain who really struggles to find positive moments in each day. Simply jotting down anything that made the day more bearable – visiting a friend, the touch of a loved one, a hot bath – will help you seek these things out in the future when you're suffering.

Play the "So-What" Game

If you're anything like me, your imagination gets carried away with any scenario in your life that holds even the slightest chance of turning out badly.

Traffic notice goes up on the motorway? *Great, I'll probably be three hours late.*

A missed call from work? *They're probably sacking me for using all the colour ink in the printer.*

Incoming email from the bank? *Someone's probably cloned my card and emptied my account. Woe is me.*

Can you relate?

Well, by now we know that stress – especially unnecessary, unwarranted, self-inflicted stress – can impact our bodies in a negative way, even amplifying painful experiences. So, what are we going to do about these harmful thinking patterns that serve no purpose but to distract us and ruin our good mood?

If you've tried to *"just stop thinking like that"*, then you'll know the harder you try, the worse it gets at times. I have been experimenting with a new method to control my own thought patterns and I have found that this really works to help me dissolve these unnecessary thoughts and avoid crippling anxiety as a result.

It's called the So-What Game and it's very simple. Every time you find a completely unfounded, disproportionate assumption about the future sneaking up on you like the ones in the example above, you need to ask yourself one question: *"So, what?"*

So, what if I AM three hours late?

In truth, it would be a minor inconvenience for the people I work with. The boss would probably understand – I'm never usually late so it's not like it's becoming a problem. Would it even be remembered tomorrow? Probably not.

So, what if I AM sacked for depleting the colour ink?

I probably wouldn't want to be in a workplace that got so twitchy about their printing costs anyway. I would have a very good case for a wrongful dismissal.

So, what if someone HAS emptied my account?

In worries like this one, the consequences are obviously greater. However, the game still works. The way you go about remedying this is by detailing in your head the *exact* step-by-step plan you'd put in place if encountering this awful situation.

You'd probably first call the bank and let them know. You might have to survive for a while without any bank cards – but most of us would have someone willing to lend us a small amount of cash for a week until it's sorted, so that should be OK. Besides, bank fraud teams are so effective nowadays there would likely be ways to prove you've been the victim of theft.

Even if you don't get your money back – are you going to die? Probably not. You'll find someone to go and live with for a while until you're back on your feet. Sell the house, get a smaller place and start fresh. You could sell your car and other belongings if you needed to.

You'd survive – and proving this to yourself is the antidote to the very crux that anxiety stems from – worrying about preservation of your life.

With this tool, it turns out there is a way that you can almost talk yourself out of this type of self-inflicted anxiety.

This technique can be a good tool to have in the toolbox for anyone struggling with low-level, day-to-day anxious thoughts. In the present day that often seems to be many of us, admittedly. I've found this tip very useful for when my thoughts start to run away with me; for the times when one feels overwhelmed by the possibility of terrible situations playing out in one's head on repeat like a broken DVD player.

I am not the first to employ this technique, as it would happen. In the ancient translated personal notes of Marcus Aurelius (Roman Emperor in 161-180AD) in the book *Meditations*, arguably the most powerful man in the world makes notes reminding himself how he must truly examine his anxieties to get to the bottom of what they really are. Once you can imagine the ultimate outcome that you fear, and you are able to say *"that really wouldn't be so bad,"* anxieties tend to abate.

Give it a try next time you feel helpless or despairing. What have you got to lose in those moments?

How to Keep the Mind Young

It is a fact that the human brain changes as we age[26]. It would be possible to see physical changes, as well as feel mental ones, in the brain of a senior when compared to the brain of someone thirty years younger. While many of these changes are unavoidable to some extent, a decline in cognition may not be necessarily inevitable.

Two of the most common mental health problems in the later stages of life are dementia and depression. The World Health Organisation[27] estimates that 5% of people over sixty suffer from dementia, while 7% suffer from depression; although these problems may be vastly underreported. Dementia is a syndrome that primarily affects the older adult but it is not a *natural* part of ageing. Depression can affect anyone of any age but the rate at which it affects the senior population is alarming.

You may have read in the media how it's possible to slow down the mental ageing process by keeping the mind active and nimble. There's a lot of truth in this claim and experts believe we should exercise the brain, just as we exercise the body. So, mental exercise is important - but how do we effectively exercise our minds to stave off the effects of ageing as much as possible?

Here are a few ways to keep your mind young and nimble in your advancing years:

• **Mental gymnastics:** Contrary to popular belief, the act of solving puzzles - such as the popular numbers game, sudoku - has never actually been shown to prevent dementia or cognitive decline. While the puzzles may improve overall cognition, they probably won't prevent dementia, a study carried out at the University of Aberdeen suggests[28]. Instead, the researchers recommend three different forms of brain exercise that may have more potential for staving off dementia: **reading, playing board games** and **playing a musical instrument**. These enjoyable yet mentally challenging tasks are hypothesised to slow down the rate of "brain atrophy" that occurs with age and help to keep the mind young.

- **Treat the body, treat the mind:** There is a wealth of evidence to suggest that exercise can act as a protective factor for both dementia and depression in advancing years[29]. People who exercise are generally happier and have better quality of life[30]. Having a healthy body really does stimulate a healthy mind, through a combination of physical and psychological factors. On the physical side, blood pressure, lipid profiles and blood sugar are all on the healthier side for people who take daily exercise[31]. Having these three markers running amok would certainly increase your risk of suffering dementia, as well as significant health events like a stroke. The fallout of an incident like a heart attack or a stroke is often long-term disability, which may lead to depression in many cases. Keep your heart healthy, your lungs in good shape and your muscles strong, and you'll be giving not just your body, but your mind as well, its best possible chance.

- **Stick the kettle on:** While the neuro-protective qualities of tea are still up for debate, there's one thing that has been shown to have a significant effect on mental health in later life; and that is your social circle. Maintaining good links between friends and family, with regular and enjoyable contact, has been proven to stimulate the mind and reduce the risks of dementia and depression alike[32]. Simply having a catch-up with a friend is enough to get your daily social quota of human contact but bonus points go to you if you engage in a fun activity with that friend too. Playing board games, taking a long walk, or going to a museum are all preferable to just sitting at home as you get the mental stimulation or exercise associated with these activities at the same time as the social aspect.

• **Avoid the deadly sins:** Smoking and drinking have been shown to be associated with an increased risk of dementia later in life, as well as a multitude of other unwanted health problems. Do your mind and body a favour and quit, or at least cut down, if you're a smoker. As for drinking, pay some attention to the government guidelines that set a clear limit for our daily alcohol intake and see how you measure up. If you regularly exceed this limit, it's probably a good idea to cut back.

• **Spend some time with Mother Nature:** There is a growing body of research, relevant to people of all ages and for a variety of health problems, that shows just how beneficial it is to spend time in the great outdoors with nature. There's evidence to show that work productivity goes up just by putting plants in offices[33]. We can significantly reduce the risk of depression just by taking long walks in the woods or on the beach[34]. Taking time to appreciate the beauty of the outdoors is a wonderful way to stay healthy in both body and mind. Be sure to schedule some time for yourself to spend in nature in the next few days and take note of how you feel after - you may find it so valuable that it becomes a non-negotiable.

Create a Healthy Habit

How do some people seemingly find it so easy to eat well, go to the gym day after day and stay in amazing shape all year round?

Are they lucky? Do they simply have good genes? Is it because they spend more money on their health than others?

I would argue that, in most cases, it's none of these things. The people who are successful with their health have simply developed healthy habits. And habits are the key to long-term success.

There is research to suggest that we have a limited amount of willpower to use in any given day[35]. Willpower is finite; by making too many decisions, we run the risk of *"willpower fatigue"*. When we reach this point of fatigue, just like having a weakened immune system; we're open to threats and are much more likely to make bad decisions that lead to poor health.

Every time you open the fridge and have to make a choice about what to eat, you're using up willpower. Every time you visit the supermarket and walk past the ice cream section, you're using up willpower. Every time you put on your trainers even though it's raining, you're using up even more of your precious willpower.

My theory is that if we have to make a decision - *"shall I, shan't I?"* - in each of these situations, we've *already* lost. There's only a certain number of times we can overcome our desire to do the easy thing before we succumb to the much more immediately pleasurable choice of staying on the sofa, ordering a takeaway or picking up that ice cream.

So, if the act of making these decisions makes it harder for us to stay healthy, what are we supposed to do? The answer is simple: *we avoid making these decisions altogether.*

At first glance, that recommendation sounds ridiculous, but if you think harder about it, it makes perfect sense. The people who are successful with making healthy decisions, day after day, do so not because they have superior willpower to us but because they put themselves into a position where they *automatically* make the right choice, without having to consider it. How do you make the right choice the automatic option? You simply have to make it far easier TO make the right choice than NOT to make it!

Let me give you some examples: if you're determined to go for a walk tomorrow morning, even when it's cold, dark and wet, make it as easy as possible for your future self by preparing the night before. Start by laying out all of your walking clothes on the end of your bed, including an extra layer if it's even colder than expected. Hide away all of your shoes, except your walking boots. Now, before you go to bed, set your alarm out of your reach when you're in bed. Tomorrow, when your alarm goes off, it'll be far easier to get up and put on your walking clothes than it will be to put them all away again and find something different to wear.

Another example I can give you represents a brilliant way to cut junk food out of your life. As it turns out, you can make healthy choices the easiest thing in the world. As humans, we have a tendency to make lifestyle choices based on convenience. This is one of the reasons why gaining weight is so easy in the first place; fattening, sugary foods are also the ones that are cheapest and easiest to get your hands on. But what would happen if you made those foods the most difficult to acquire, and healthier foods the most *convenient* option? Do you think you'd make better choices?

One way to do this is to be sure to eat a satiating meal before you go for your weekly shop (we make worse food purchasing decisions when hungry), so you find it much easier to buy only healthy foods and leave your usual temptations on the shelves. Even better, write a strict list before you go, foregoing any junk food. When you get home, discard or ask a friend to take the sugary, fattening foods that currently live in your kitchen and pantry so you're left with nothing in the house except healthy food. The third part of this process is to ensure you make a small amount extra of any healthy meal and store it in the fridge, so you have emergency snacks should you get hungry between meals.

When the cravings arise - and they will - you'll have a choice; eat the pre-prepared healthy food… or get your wallet, get in your car, drive all the way to the shop and buy a sugary snack. Eight to nine times out of ten, you'll likely opt for the healthier choice out of sheer convenience. In this way, you don't even need to think of this process as "being on a diet". You're still allowed the naughty food, after all; you just have to work a little harder for it!

By making the right choice the *default* choice, you make it much easier for your brain to shortcut the decision making process. These little choices all add up, and it gets easier as time goes on. After you make the right choice hundreds of times in a row, a habit is formed. And when a habit is formed, it becomes more effort to go against your healthy habit than it does to follow it from here on.

Conclusion

The human body is a complex and wonderful creation. The sheer astonishing scale of the tiny but significant chemical reactions that occur within our bodies every day to keep us alive is enough to spend a lifetime wondering over. Within this plethora of reactions is the human ability to feel pain. While it may not feel like a blessing at times, pain is as valuable and important a sensation as touch, smell or taste.

The power of pain

Pain guides us every single day of our lives.

Pain is the reason you instinctively react to pull your hand away from a knife blade. Pain is the driving force behind the muscles in your ankle contracting to prevent an ankle sprain, before your consciousness can even begin to process that action.

And on another level, emotional pain moves us to take action. It motivates us to make changes. If we didn't get uncomfortable sometimes, we wouldn't have the drive to accomplish anything significant.

Without certain types of pain, we would not survive for long. However, pain isn't always necessary. In this book, I've tried to provide you with some solutions to nagging, painful problems that get in the way of living life to its fullest. Hopefully, you've learned something along the way that you can now apply to your own life.

If you aren't suffering from a painful problem, I hope you've still found great value in the recommendations I've discovered and presented to you about how we should be living to prolong life as best we can. We only get one chance at this game of life, and making small daily actions into healthy habits is the way to ensure your health for the years ahead of you.

Not just the physical

Of course, as we've discussed in this book, it isn't just the health of your body that you need to pay attention to. The mind is just as important, and strategies to improve your mental health and wellbeing are as valuable as physical exercise when it comes to staying fit and able in your advancing years.

My challenge to you upon completion of this book is to simply remain aware of the areas of your body and mind that might need a little work to remain healthy as you grow older. Did you struggle to complete the *Nine at Ninety*? Do you have aches or pains that haven't resolved over the last few months? Are you feeling lonely or in need of some mental stimulation? If you answered "yes" to any of these questions, you know exactly where you need to start in order to get and stay physically and mentally healthy.

An important thing to remember as you spend a bit more time working on your health is that you're not alone in this. There are people who have dedicated their careers to helping others achieve these (often overwhelming) goals of becoming or staying healthy despite their years working against them. I am one of such people. So, if you're in Surrey and would like a helping hand, you'd be more than welcome to stop by for a chat and a coffee where we can talk about exactly what we need to do to get you fit, healthy and mobile again.

Simply head to **https://ht-physio.co.uk** if you'd like to learn more about how you can get some help to achieve your goals.

If you're not in my area, but would still like some help, it's worth speaking to a few local professionals about how they can help and, most importantly, the kind of results they have achieved for others before. Don't be afraid to "put them on trial" - it's the only way you'll be able to tell if they have the skills and capabilities to help you reach your goals.

Biggest take home message

If I had to distil the take home message from this book down to one sentence, it would be this: *Please don't feel as though you have to accept aches, pains, poor mobility, "slowing down", becoming lonely and missing out on the things you love as just a part of getting older!*

There is no need for it to be that way for most people reading this, and there are usually things that can be done to improve your situation, even if you've initially been told you just need to "accept it" as a fact of life. I am an advocate for second opinions; it's something we try to do for people every day in my clinic. So, if nothing else, please take the hope that I'm trying to pass onto you from these pages that growing older doesn't have to represent a slow decline in health and mobility. People regularly come into my clinic and say *"it's no fun getting old,"* but I like to encourage them to see the positives that they can take from their advancing years. Experience, wisdom and patience are all virtues that we gain with each passing year and I'm sure you are no different.

One of the greatest gifts you can give to yourself in your fifties and beyond is the gift of physical activity. Staying active has been shown to protect your heart, muscles and even your brain. It's a common occurrence to hear a doctor remark that if there was a pill that could give us the benefits of exercise, people would be queuing round the corner to get a prescription. Luckily, we don't need to wait until a wonder-drug is invented when there are so many different forms of exercise and activity that are readily available to us; just pick one that works for you. Summoning the willpower to get started is genuinely the biggest hurdle but the more you flex that hypothetical muscle, the stronger it gets. Keep making the right choices for your body, day after day, and the little decisions all add up.

As for following diets and nutrition plans, don't over-complicate it. Try to make better choices, one by one, and take advantage of our tendencies to take the most convenient option we have available to us (discussed on page 296). If you're looking to shed a few pounds, this may involve putting obstacles in the way between you and junk food.

Armed with the information and guidance in this book, you should have a better chance of remaining healthy and injury-free, which will directly improve your quality of life and the lives of your family. One thing that my clients report worrying about perhaps more than anything else is that their family may have to suffer in order to take care of them as they become sick or less mobile. By staying fit, well and injury-free, you'll not only be giving yourself an incredible gift, but you'll also be doing the same for your family. Imagine having a few extra years to play with the grandchildren that you otherwise wouldn't have had; can you put a price on that?

My Final Gift To You

I hope you'll consider downloading my free gift to you with this book: *The Top 5 Exercises for Over-50's Who Want to Remain Strong, Mobile & Active.* I've laid out the benefits of resistance training on page 218, and this free downloadable guide will show you the way to achieve those benefits in later life. It is quite literally a roadmap to achieving strength, mobility and health. It just needs a little effort on your part but I know you'll be able to get there. You can find this valuable guide and take it for free at:

https://ht-physio.co.uk/guide/

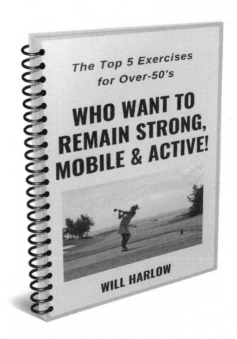

About The Author

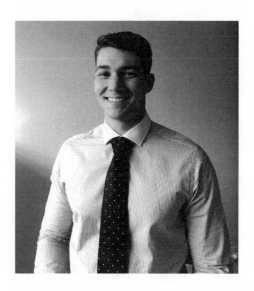

Will Harlow is a physiotherapist with a mission to help over-fifties stay mobile, healthy and active, without the use of pain pills or surgery.

He graduated from Brunel University in 2015, where he received a first-class masters degree in physiotherapy. He then went on to work in the NHS as a junior, senior and team leader. He also enjoyed a stint working in professional football for the biggest football club on the South Coast of England. He authored a book dedicated to helping people recover from sciatica in 2018 called *The 7 Steps to Overcome Sciatica.*

He now works and lives in Surrey, running his private physiotherapy practice, HT Physio, in Farnham.

In his spare time, Will enjoys sport, travel and collecting funk, soul and disco records. He lives with his girlfriend, Bryony, and their cat, Pablo.

References

CRACKING THE FUNDAMENTALS

[1] Matthews, C.E., Moore, S.C., Arem, H., Cook, M.B., Trabert, B., Hakansson, N., Larsson, S.C., Wolk, A., Gapstur, S.M., Lynch, B.M., Milne, R.L., Freedman, N.D., Huang, W.Y., Berrington de Golzalez, A., Kitahara, C.M., Linet, M.S., Shiroma, E.J., Sandin, S., Pavel, A.V., Lee, I.M. (2019). Amount and intensity of leisure-time physical activity and lower cancer risk. *Journal of Clinical Oncology*. [ePub ahead of print].

[2] Wange, R., Holsinger, R.M.D. (2018). Exercise-induced brain-derived neurotrophic factor expression: therapeutic implications for Alzheimer's dementia. *Ageing Research Review*. **48**. 109-121.

HEAD, NECK & SHOULDERS

[1] Shaik, M.M., Gan, S.H. (2015). Vitamin supplementation as possible prophylactic treatment against migraine with aura and menstrual migraine. *Biomed Res Int*. Online pub Feb 2015.

[2] Wang, K., Ho, V., Hunter-Smith, D.J., Beh, P.S., Smith, K.M., Weber, A.B. Risk factors in idiopathic adhesive capsulitis: a case control study. *J Shoulder Elbow Surg*. 2013; **22**(7):e24–e29.

[3] Malavolta, E.A., Gracitelli, M.E.C., Ribeiro Pinto, G.M., Freire da Silveira, A.Z., Assunção, J.H., Ferreira Neto, A.A.. Asian ethnicity: a risk factor for adhesive capsulitis?. *Rev Bras Ortop*. 2018; **53**(5):602–606.

[4] Franz, A., Klose, M., Beitzel, K. 2019. Conservative treatment of frozen shoulder. *Unfallchirurg*. **122**(12). 934-940.

[5] Pieters, L., Lewis, J., Kuppens, K., Jochems, J., Bruijstens, T., Joossens, L., Struyf, F. (2019). An update of systematic reviews examining the effectiveness of conservative physiotherapy interventions for subacromial shoulder pain. *Journal of Orthopaedics and Sports Physical Therapy*. 1-33.

[6] Lawrence, R.L., Moutzouros, V., Bey, M.J. (2019). Asymptomatic rotator cuff tears. *JBJS Rev.* **7**(6). 9.

[7] Horsley, I., Herrington, L., Hoyle, R., Prescott, E., Bellamy, N. (2016). Do changes in hand grip strength correlate with shoulder rotator cuff function? *Shoulder Elbow.* **8** (2). 124-129.

WRISTS, ELBOWS & HANDS

[1] van den Heuvel, S.G., de Looze, M.O., Hildebrandt, V.H., The, K.H. (2003). Effects of software programs stimulating regular breaks and exercises on work-related neck and upper-limb disorders. *Scand J Work Environ Health.* **29**(2). 106-116.

[2] Kim, T.N., Choi, K.M. Sarcopenia: definition, epidemiology, and pathophysiology. *J Bone Metab.* 2013; **20**(1):1-10.

[3] Moore, D.R. Keeping older muscle "young" through dietary protein and physical activity. *Adv Nutr.* 2014; **5**(5). 599-607.

BACK PAIN & SCIATICA

[1] National Institute of Neurological Disorders and Stroke https://www.ninds.nih.gov/ Disorders/Patient-Caregiver-Education/Fact-Sheets/Low-Back-Pain-Fact-Sheet

[2] Eshed, I., Lidar, M. (2017). MRI Findings of the Sacroiliac Joints in Patients with Low Back Pain: Alternative Diagnosis to Inflammatory Sacroiliitis. *Isr Med Assoc J.* **19**(11). 666-669.

[3] Assaker, R., Zairi, F. (2015). Failed back surgery syndrome: to re-operate or not to re-operate? A retrospective review of patient selection and failures. *Neurochirurgie.* **61**. 77-82.

[4] Brinjikji, W., Luetmer, P.H., Comstock, B., et al. Systematic literature review of imaging features of spinal degeneration in asymptomatic populations. *AJNR Am J Neuroradiol.* 2015; **36**(4):811–816.

[5] Berthelot, J.M., Laredo, J.D., Darrieutort-Laffite, C., Maugars, Y. (2018) Stretching of roots contributes to the pathophysiology of radiculopathies. *Joint Bone Spine.* **85**(1): 41-45

[6] Strauss, A.T., Parr, A.J., Desmond, D.J., Vargas, A.T., Baker, R.T. (2019). The effect of total motion release on functional movement screen composite scores: A randomised controlled trial. *Journal of Sports Rehabilitation*. Dec 2019. 1-9.

[7] Sheahan, P.J., Diesbourg, T.L., Fischer, S.L. (2016). The effect of rest break schedule on acute low back pain development in pain and non-pain developers during seated work. *Appl Ergon*. **53**. 64-70.

[8] Daneshmandi H, Choobineh A, Ghaem H, Karimi M. Adverse Effects of Prolonged Sitting Behavior on the General Health of Office Workers. *J Lifestyle Med*. 2017; **7**(2): 69–75.

[9] Szczygiel, E., Zielonka, K., Metel, S., Golec, J. (2017). Musculo-skeletal and pulmonary effects of sitting position - a systematic review. *Ann Agric Environ Med*. **24**(1). 8-12.

[10] De Blaiser, C., Roosen, P., Willems, T., Danneels, L., Bossche, L.V., De Ridder, R. (2018). Is core stability a risk factor for lower extremity injuries in an athletic population? A systematic review. *Phys Ther Sport*. **30**. 48-56.

[11] Kendall, J.C., Bird, A.Z., Azari, M.F. (2014). Foot posture, leg length discrepancy and low back pain — their relationship and clinical management using foot orthoses — an overview. *Foot (Edinburgh)*. **24**(2). 75-80.

[12] Resende, R.A., Pinheiro, L.S.P., Ocarina, J.M. (2019). Effects of foot pronation on the lower limb sagittal plane biomechanics during gait. *Gait Posture*. **68**. 130-135.

[13] Unver, B., Erdem, E.U., Akbas, E. (2019). Effects of short-foot exercises on foot posture, pain, disability, and plantar pressure in pen planus. *Journal of Sports Rehabilitation*. **16**. 1-5.

HIPS & KNEES

1 Alaia, M.J., Khatib, O., Shah, M., A Bosco, J., M Jazrawi, L., Strauss, E.J. (2015). The utility of plan radiographs in the initial evaluation of knee pain amongst sports medicine patients. *Knee Surg Sports Traumatol Arthrosc*. **23**(8). 2213-2217.

2 de Oliveira Silva, D., Barton, C., Crossley, K., Waiteman, M., Taborda, B., Ferreira, A.S., Azevedo, F.M. (2018). Implications of knee crepitus to the overall clinical presentation of women with and without patellofemoral pain. *Physical Therapy in Sport*. **33**. 89-95.

3 Glaviano, N.R., Saliba, S. (2019). Differences in gluteal and quadriceps muscle activation during weight-bearing exercises between female subjects with and without patellofemoral pain. *Journal of Strength and Conditioning Research.* [epub ahead of print].

4 Schiphof, D., van Middelkoop, M., de Klerk, B.M., Oei, E.H., Hofman, A., Koes, B.W., Weinans, H., Bierma-Zeinstra, S.M. (2014). Crepitus is a first indication of patellofemoral osteoarthritis (and not of tibiofemoral arthritis). *Osteoarthritis Cartilage.* **22**(5). 631-638.

5 Mun, F., Suh, S.W., Park, H.J., Choi, A. (2015). Kinematic relationship between rotation of lumbar spine and hip joints during golf swing in professional golfers. *Biomed Eng Online.* **14.** 41.

6 MacDonald, K.V., Sanmartin, C., Langlois, K., Marshall, D.A. (2014). Symptom onset, diagnosis and management of osteoarthritis. *Health Rep.* **25**(9). 10-17.

7 Klassbo, M., Harms-Ringdahl, K., Larsson, G. (2003). Examination of passive ROM and capsular patterns in the hip. *Physiother Res Int.* **8**(1). 1-12.

8 Park, K.N., Kwon, O.Y., Yi, C.H., Cynn, H.S., Weon, J.H., Kim, T.H., Choi, H.S. (2016). Effects of motor control exercise vs muscle stretching exercise on reducing compensatory lumbopelvic motions and low back pain: a randomised trial. *J Manipulative Physiol Ther.* **39**(8). 576-585.

9 Jibri, Z., Jamieson, P., Rakhra, K.S., Sampaio, M.L., Dervin, G. (2019). Patellar maltracking: an update on the diagnosis and treatment strategies. *Insights Imaging.* **10**(1). 65.

10 Li, J.S., Tsai, T.Y., Clancy, M.M., Li, G., Lewis, C.L., Felson, D.T. (2019). Weight loss changed gait kinematics in individuals with obesity and knee pain. *Gait Posture.* **68.** 461-465.

11 Sherrington, C., Tiedemann, A. (2015). Physiotherapy in the prevention of falls in older people. *Journal of Physiotherapy.* **61.** 54-60.

12 Negendank, W.G., Fernandez-Madrid, F.R., Heilbrun, L.K., Teitge, R.A. (1990). Magnetic resonance imaging of meniscal degeneration in asymptomatic knees. *J Orthop Res.* **8**(3). 311-320.

13 Jin, X., Ding, C., Wang, X., Antony, B., Laslett, L.L., Blizzard, L., Cicuttini, F., Jones, G. (2016). Longitudinal associations between adiposity and change in knee pain: Tasmanian older adult cohort study. *Semin Arthritis Rheum.* **45**(5). 564-569.

14 Hicks-Little, C.A., Peindl, R.D., Hubbard-Turner, T.J., Cordova, M.L. (2016). The relationship between early-stage knee osteoarthritis and lower-extremity alignment, joint

laxity, and subjective scores of pain, stiffness and function. *J Sport Rehabil.* **25**(3). 213-218.

15 Lee, J.Y., Han, K., McAlindon, T.E., Park, Y.G., Park, S.H. (2018). Lower leg muscle mass relates to knee pain in patients with knee osteoarthritis. *Int J Rheum Dis.* **21**(1). 126-133.

16 Guedes, V., Castro, J.P., Brito, I. (2018). Topical capsaicin for pain in osteoarthritis: A literature review. *Rheumatol Clin.* **14**(1). 40-45.

17 Hurley M, Dickson K, Hallett R, et al. Exercise interventions and patient beliefs for people with hip, knee or hip and knee osteoarthritis: a mixed methods review. *Cochrane Database Syst Rev.* 2018; 4(4):CD010842. Published 2018 Apr 17.

18 Torres, A., Fernandez-Fairen, M., Sueiro-Fernandez, J. (2018). Greater trochanteric pain syndrome and gluteus medius and minibus tendinosis: nonsurgical treatment. *Pain Management.* **8**(1). 45-55.

19 Ganderton, C., Pizzari, T., Harle, T., Cook, J., Semciw, A. (2017). A comparison of gluteus medius, gluteus minimus and tensor fascia latae muscle activation during gait in post-menopausal women with and without greater trochanteric pain syndrome. *J Electromyogr Kinesiol.* **33**. 39-47.

20 Paluska, S.A., McKeag, D.B. (2000). Knee braces: current evidence and clinical recommendations for their use. *American Family Physician.* **61**(2). 411-418.

21 Jensen, S.B., Henriksen, M., Aaboe, J., Hansen, L., Simonsen, E.B., Alkjaer, T. (2010). Is it possible to reduce the knee joint compression force during level walking with hiking poles? *Scandinavian Journal of Medicine & Science in Sports.* **21**(6). 195-200.

FEET & ANKLES

1 de Jonge S, van den Berg C, de Vos RJ, *et al*Incidence of midportion Achilles tendinopathy in the general population. *British Journal of Sports Medicine.* 2011;**45**:1026-1028.

2 Chang HJ, Burke AE, Glass RM. Achilles Tendinopathy. *JAMA.* 2010;**303**(2):188.

3 Roche, A.J., Calder, J.D.F. (2013). Achilles tendinopathy: A review of the current concepts of treatment. *Bone Joint Journal.* **95**. 1299-1307.

4 Redmond, A.C., Crane, Y.Z. & Menz, H.B. 2008. Normative values for the Foot Posture Index. *J Foot Ankle Res* **1**, 6.

5 Gross, K.D., Felson, D.T., Niu, J., Hunter, D.J., Guermazi, A., Roemer, F.W., Dufour, A.B., Gensure, R.H. and Hannan, M.T. (2011), Association of flat feet with knee pain and cartilage damage in older adults. *Arthritis Care Res,* **63**: 937-944.

6 Latey, P.J., Burns, J., Hiller, C. *et al.* Relationship between intrinsic foot muscle weakness and pain: a systematic review. *J Foot Ankle Res* **7,** 51.

7 Hertel, J. Functional instability following lateral ankle sprain. *Sports Med* (2000) **29**: 361.

8 Kibler, W. B., Goldberg, C., & Chandler, T. J. (1991). Functional biomechanical deficits in running athletes with plantar fasciitis. *The American Journal of Sports Medicine, 19*(1), 66–71.

9 Torg JS, Pavlov H, Torg E. Overuse injuries in sport: the foot. *Clinics in Sports Medicine.* 1987 Apr; **6**(2):291-320.

10 McClinton, S., Collazo, C., Vincent, E., Vardaxis, V. (2016). Impaired Foot Plantar Flexor Muscle Performance in Individuals With Plantar Heel Pain and Association With Foot Orthosis Use. *Journal of Orthopaedic & Sports Physical Therapy,* 2016 :**46** (8) : 681–688.

11 Cychosz CC, Phisitkul P, Belatti DA, Glazebrook MA, DiGiovanni CW. Gastrocnemius recession for foot and ankle conditions in adults: Evidence-based recommendations. *Foot Ankle Surg.* 2015 Jun;**21**(2):77-85.

12 Bolívar YA, Munuera PV, Padillo JP. Relationship between tightness of the posterior muscles of the lower limb and plantar fasciitis. Foot Ankle Int. 2013 Jan;34(1): 42-8.

13 Clinghan R, Arnold GP, Drew TS, Cochrane LA, Abboud RJ. Do you get value for money when you buy an expensive pair of running shoes? *Br J Sports Med.* 2008 Mar; **42**(3):189-93.

WHOLE BODY HEALTH

1 Marsolais D, Frenette J. Inflammation and tendon healing. *Medecine Sciences : M/ S.* 2005 Feb; **21**(2):181-186.

2 Izaola O, de Luis D, Sajoux I, Domingo JC, Vidal M. Inflammation and obesity (lipoinflammation). *Nutr Hosp.* 2015 Jun **1;31**(6):2352-8.

3 Butkowski EG, Jelinek HF. Hyperglycaemia, oxidative stress and inflammatory markers. *Redox Rep.* 2017 Nov; **22**(6):257-264.

4 Li M, van Esch BCAM, Wagenaar GTM, Garssen J, Folkerts G, Henricks PAJ. Pro- and anti-inflammatory effects of short chain fatty acids on immune and endothelial cells. *Eur J Pharmacol.* 2018 Jul 15; **831**:52-59.

5 Tibuakuu M, Kamimura D, Kianoush S, DeFilippis AP, Al Rifai M, Reynolds LM, White WB, Butler KR, Mosley TH, Turner ST, Kullo IJ, Hall ME, Blaha MJ. The association between cigarette smoking and inflammation: The Genetic Epidemiology Network of Arteriopathy (GENOA) study. *PLoS One.* 2017 Sep 18;12(9).

6 Lancaster T, Stead LF. Individual behavioural counselling for smoking cessation. Cochrane Database of Systematic Reviews 2017, Issue 3. Art. No.: CD001292.

7 Imhof, A., Froehlich, M., Brenner, H., Boeing, H., Pepys, M.B., Koenig, W. Effect of alcohol consumption on systemic markers of inflammation. *The Lancet.* **357** (9258). 2001, Pages 763-767.

8 Elks, C.M. & Francis. Central adiposity, systemic inflammation, and the metabolic syndrome. *J. Curr Hypertens Rep* (2010) **12**: 99.

9 Gunathilake KDPP, Ranaweera KKDS, Rupasinghe HPV. In Vitro Anti-Inflammatory Properties of Selected Green Leafy Vegetables. Biomedicines. 2018 Nov 19;6(4). pii: E107.

10 Korrapati D, Jeyakumar SM, Putcha UK, Mendu VR, Ponday LR, Acharya V, Koppala SR, Vajreswari A. Coconut oil consumption improves fat-free mass, plasma HDL-cholesterol and insulin sensitivity in healthy men with normal BMI compared to peanut oil. Clin Nutr. 2019 Dec;38(6):2889-2899.

11 Wongwarawipat T, Papageorgiou N, Bertsias D, Siasos G, Tousoulis D. Olive Oil-related Anti-inflammatory Effects on Atherosclerosis: Potential Clinical Implications. *Endocr Metab Immune Disord Drug Targets.* 2018; **18**(1):51-62.

12 Artemis P. Simopoulos (2002) Omega-3 Fatty Acids in Inflammation and Autoimmune Diseases, *Journal of the American College of Nutrition*, 21:6, 495-505.

13 https://www.bda.uk.com/foodfacts/omega3.pdf

14 Lisa S. McAnulty, David C. Nieman, Charles L. Dumke, Lesli A. Shooter, Dru A. Henson, Alan C. Utter, Ginger Milne, Steven R. McAnulty. Effect of blueberry ingestion on natural killer cell counts, oxidative stress, and inflammation prior to and after 2.5 h of running. Applied Physiology, Nutrition, and Metabolism, 2011, 36:976-984,

15 Murphy, M.H., Nevill, A.M., Neville, C., Biddle, S., Hardman, A.E. 2002. Accumulating brisk walking for fitness, cardiovascular risk, and psychological health. Med. Sci. Sports Exerc., Vol. 34, No. 9, pp. 1468–1474.

16 Guthrie, J.R., Dennerstein, L., Taffe, J.R., Ebeling, P.R., Randolph, J.F., Burger, H.G., Wark, J.D. Central abdominal fat and endogenous hormones during the menopausal transition, *Fertility and Sterility.* **79** (6), 2003, Pages 1335-1340.

17 Dumoulin C, Hay–Smith EJC, Mac Habée–Séguin G. Pelvic floor muscle training versus no treatment, or inactive control treatments, for urinary incontinence in women. Cochrane Database of Systematic Reviews 2014, Issue 5.

18 John E. Morley, Fran E. Kaiser, Horace M. Perry, Ping Patrick, Patricia M.K. Morley, Patricia M. Stauber, Bruno Vellas, Richard N. Baumgartner, Phillip J. Garry. Longitudinal changes in testosterone, luteinizing hormone, and follicle-stimulating hormone in healthy older men. *Metabolism.* **46** (4). 1997. Pages 410-413.

19 Molly M. Shores, Nicholas L. Smith, Christopher W. Forsberg, Bradley D. Anawalt, Alvin M. Matsumoto, Testosterone Treatment and Mortality in Men with Low Testosterone Levels, *The Journal of Clinical Endocrinology & Metabolism*, Volume 97, Issue 6, 1 June 2012, Pages 2050–2058.

20 S. Pilz, S. Frisch, H. Koertke, J. Kuhn, J. Dreier, B. Obermayer-Pietsch, E. Wehr, A. Zittermann. Effect of Vitamin D Supplementation on Testosterone Levels in Men. Horm Metab Res 2011; 43(3): 223-225.

21 J MacLaughlin, M F Holick. Aging decreases the capacity of human skin to produce vitamin D3. *J Clin Invest.* 1985;76(4):1536-1538.

22 Thomas J. Littlejohns, William E. Henley, Iain A. Lang, Cedric Annweiler, Olivier Beauchet, Paulo H.M. Chaves, Linda Fried, Bryan R. Kestenbaum, Lewis H. Kuller, Kenneth M. Langa, Oscar L. Lopez, Katarina Kos, Maya Soni, David J. Llewellyn. Vitamin D and the risk of dementia and Alzheimer disease. Neurology Sep 2014, 83 (10) 920-928.

23 William J. Kraemer, Keijo Häkkinen, Robert U. Newton, Bradley C. Nindl, Jeff S. Volek, Matthew McCormick, Lincoln A. Gotshalk, Scott E. Gordon, Steven J. Fleck, Wayne W. Campbell, Margot Putukian, and William J. Evans. Effects of heavy-resistance training on hormonal response patterns in younger vs. older men. *Journal of Applied Physiology* 1999 **87**:3, 982-992.

24 Hunter, G.R., McCarthy, J.P. & Bamman, M.M. Effects of Resistance Training on Older Adults. *Sports Med* **34,** 329–348 (2004).

25 Layne, J.E., Nelson, M.E. 1999. The effects of progressive resistance training on bone density: a review. *Medicine & Science in Sports & Exercise.* **31**(1). 25-30.

26 Susan Hudec and Pauline Camacho (*2013*) Secondary Causes of Osteoporosis. Endocrine Practice: January 2013, Vol. 19, No. 1, pp. 120-128.

27 Melton, L.J., III, Chrischilles, E.A., Cooper, C., Lane, A.W. and Riggs, B.L. (2005), How Many Women Have Osteoporosis?. J Bone Miner Res, 20: 886-892.

28 Pacifici, R. (1996), Estrogen, cytokines, and pathogenesis of postmenopausal osteoporosis. J Bone Miner Res, 11: 1043-1051.

29 Michael F Holick, Vitamin D: importance in the prevention of cancers, type 1 diabetes, heart disease, and osteoporosis, *The American Journal of Clinical Nutrition*, Volume 79, Issue 3, March 2004, Pages 362–371.

30 Anne B. Newman, Varant Kupelian, Marjolein Visser, Eleanor M. Simonsick, Bret H. Goodpaster, Stephen B. Kritchevsky, Frances A. Tylavsky, Susan M. Rubin, Tamara B. Harris, on Behalf of the Health, Aging and Body Composition Study Investigators, Strength, But Not Muscle Mass, Is Associated With Mortality in the Health, Aging and Body Composition Study Cohort, *The Journals of Gerontology: Series A*, Volume 61, Issue 1, January 2006, Pages 72–77.

31 C. WICKHAM, C. COOPER, B. M. MARGETTS, D. J. P. BARKER, Muscle Strength, Activity, Housing and the Risk of Falls in Elderly People, *Age and Ageing*, Volume 18, Issue 1, January 1989, Pages 47–51.

32 Schilke, Joyce M.; Johnson, Glen O.; Housh, Terry J.; O'Dell, James R. Effects of Muscle-Strength Training on the Functional Status of Patients with Osteoarthritis of the Knee Joint Nursing Research: March-April 1996 - Volume 45 - Issue 2 - p 68-72

33 J J Cunningham, Body composition and resting metabolic rate: the myth of feminine metabolism, *The American Journal of Clinical Nutrition*, Volume 36, Issue 4, October 1982, Pages 721–726.

34 Lachman, M. E., Neupert, S. D., Bertrand, R., & Jette, A. M. (2006). The Effects of Strength Training on Memory in Older Adults, *Journal of Aging and Physical Activity*, *14*(1), 59-73.

35 Hickson RC, Rosenkoetter MA, Brown MM. Strength training effects on aerobic power and short-term endurance. Medicine and Science in Sports and Exercise. 1980 ; 12(5):336-339.

36 James Rainville, Carol Hartigan, Eugenio Martinez, Janet Limke, Cristin Jouve, Mark Finno, Exercise as a treatment for chronic low back pain, The Spine Journal, Volume 4, Issue 1, 2004, Pages 106-115.

37 O'Connor, P. J., Herring, M. P., & Caravalho, A. (2010). Mental Health Benefits of Strength Training in Adults. *American Journal of Lifestyle Medicine*, *4*(5), 377–396.

38 Mayer F, Scharhag-Rosenberger F, Carlsohn A, et al.: The intensity and effects of strength training in the elderly. Dtsch Arztebl Int 2011; 108(21): 359–64.

39 Sawitzke AD, Shi H, Finco MF, Dunlop DD, Harris CL, Singer NG, Bradley JD, Silver D, Jackson CG, Lane NE, Oddis CV, Wolfe F, Lisse J, Furst DE, Bingham CO, Reda DJ, Moskowitz RW, Williams HJ, Clegg DO. Clinical efficacy and safety of glucosamine, chondroitin sulphate, their combination, celecoxib or placebo taken to treat osteoarthritis of the knee: 2-year results from GAIT. Ann Rheum Dis. 2010; **69**(8): 1459-64.

40 Yves Henrotin, Marc Marty, Ali Mobasheri, What is the current status of chondroitin sulfate and glucosamine for the treatment of knee osteoarthritis?, Maturitas, Volume 78, Issue 3, 2014, Pages 184-187.

41 https://www.theguardian.com/lifeandstyle/2017/sep/24/why-lack-of-sleep-health-worst-enemy-matthew-walker-why-we-sleep

42 Chellappa, S.L., Steiner, R., Oelhafen, P., Lang, D., Götz, T., Krebs, J. and Cajochen, C. (2013), Acute exposure to evening blue–enriched light impacts on human sleep. J Sleep Res, 22: 573-580.

43 Patricia J. Murphy, Scott S. Campbell, Nighttime Drop in Body Temperature: A Physiological Trigger for Sleep Onset?, *Sleep*, Volume 20, Issue 7, July 1997, Pages 505–511,

44 Mertens, I.L. and van, Gaal, L.F. (2000), Overweight, Obesity, and Blood Pressure: The Effects of Modest Weight Reduction. Obesity Research, 8: 270-278.

45 Yekeen, L.A., Sanusi, R.A., Ketiku, A.O. (2003). Prevalence of obesity and high level of cholesterol in hypertension. *African Journal of Biomedical Research*. **6**. 129-132.

46 Lu Qi, Peter Kraft, David J. Hunter, Frank B. Hu, The common obesity variant near *MC4R* gene is associated with higher intakes of total energy and dietary fat, weight change and diabetes risk in women, *Human Molecular Genetics*, Volume 17, Issue 22, 15 November 2008, Pages 3502–3508.

47 Wolin, K.Y., Carson, K. and Colditz, G.A. (2010), Obesity and Cancer. The Oncologist, 15: 556-565.

48 Suk, S-H., Sacco, R.L., Boden-Albala, B., Cheun, J.F., Pittman, J.G., Elkind, M.S., Paik, M.C. (2003). Abdominal obesity and risk of ischemic stroke: The northern Manhattan stroke study. *Stroke*. **23**. 1586-1592.

49 Marks, R. (2007), Obesity Profiles with Knee Osteoarthritis: Correlation with Pain, Disability, Disease Progression. Obesity, 15: 1867-1874.

50 Kristin Anderson, Rose L. Hamm, Factors That Impair Wound Healing, Journal of the American College of Clinical Wound Specialists, Volume 4, Issue 4, 2012, Pages 84-91.

51 Malik, V.S., Popkin, B.M., Bray, G.A., Despres, J-P., Hu, F.B. (2010). Sugar-sweetened beverages, obesity, type 2 diabetes mellitus, and cardiovascular disease risk. *Circulation.* **121**. 1356-1364.

52 Grover, Steven A et al. 2015. Years of life lost and healthy life-years lost from diabetes and cardiovascular disease in overweight and obese people: a modelling study. The Lancet Diabetes & Endocrinology, Volume 3, Issue 2, 114 - 122.

53 E. T. Poehlman, M. I. Goran, A. W. Gardner, P. A. Ades, P. J. Arciero, S. M. Katzman-Rooks, S. M. Montgomery, M. J. Toth, and P. T. Sutherland. Determinants of decline in resting metabolic rate in aging females. American Journal of Physiology-Endocrinology and Metabolism. 1993 264:3, E450-E455.

54 Helge, J.W. Adaptation to a Fat-Rich Diet. *Sports Med* **30**, 347–357 (2000).

55 https://www.gov.uk/government/news/behind-the-headlines-calorie-guidelines-remain-unchanged

56 Passmore, R. (1956). Daily energy expenditure by man. Proceedings of the Nutrition Society, 15(1), 83-89.

57 https://www.gov.uk/government/publications/the-eatwell-guide

58 Katiyar, S.K. and Mukhtar, H. (1997), Tea antioxidants in cancer. Chemoprevention. J. Cell. Biochem., 67: 59-67.

59 Imran A, Butt MS, Arshad MS, Arshad MU, Saeed F, Sohaib M, Munir R. Exploring the potential of black tea based flavonoids against hyperlipidemia related disorders. Lipids Health Dis. 2018 Mar 27;17(1):57.

60 Fujita H, Yamagami T. Antihypercholesterolemic effect of Chinese black tea extract in human subjects with borderline hypercholesterolemia. Nutr Res. 2008 Jul; 28(7):450-6.

61 Larsson SC, Virtamo J, Wolk A. Black tea consumption and risk of stroke in women and men. Ann Epidemiol. 2013 Mar;23(3):157-60.

62 Arab L, Liu W, Elashoff D. Green and black tea consumption and risk of stroke: a meta-analysis. Stroke. 2009 May;40(5):1786-92.

63 Maia L, de Mendonça A. Does caffeine intake protect from Alzheimer's disease? Eur J Neurol. 2002 Jul;9(4):377-82.

64 Hedström AK, Mowry EM, Gianfrancesco MA, et al High consumption of coffee is associated with decreased multiple sclerosis risk; results from two independent studies Journal of Neurology, Neurosurgery & Psychiatry 2016;87:454-460.

65 Coffee Consumption and the Risk of Colorectal Cancer Stephanie L. Schmit, Hedy S. Rennert, Gad Rennert and Stephen B. Gruber Cancer Epidemiol Biomarkers Prev April 1 2016 (25) (4) 634-639

66 Park S, Freedman ND, Haiman CA, et al. Association of Coffee Consumption With Total and Cause-Specific Mortality Among Nonwhite Populations. Ann Intern Med. 2017;167:228–235.

67 Bassett DR Jr, Toth LP, LaMunion SR, Crouter SE. Step Counting: A Review of Measurement Considerations and Health-Related Applications. Sports Med. 2017 Jul; 47(7):1303-1315.

68 Bennett GG, Wolin KY, Puleo E, Emmons KM. Pedometer-determined physical activity among multiethnic low-income housing residents. Med Sci Sports Exerc. 2006;38(4):768–773.

69 https://www.bbc.co.uk/news/health-42864061

70 Ohori T., Nozawa T., Ihori H., et al. Effect of repeated sauna treatment on exercise tolerance and endothelial function in patients with chronic heart failure. American Journal of Cardiology. 2012;109(1):100–104.

71 Beever R. The effects of repeated thermal therapy on quality of life in patients with type II diabetes mellitus. The Journal of Alternative and Complementary Medicine. 2010;16(6):677–681.

72 Shinsato T., Miyata M., Kubozono T., et al. Waon therapy mobilizes CD34+ cells and improves peripheral arterial disease. Journal of Cardiology. 2010;56(3):361–366.

73 Mark F. McCarty, Jorge Barroso-Aranda, Francisco Contreras, Regular thermal therapy may promote insulin sensitivity while boosting expression of endothelial nitric oxide synthase – Effects comparable to those of exercise training, Medical Hypotheses, Volume 73, Issue 1, 2009, Pages 103-105,

74 Laukkanen T., Kunutsor S., Kauhanen J., Laukkanen J. A. Sauna bathing is inversely associated with dementia and Alzheimer's disease in middle-aged Finnish men. Age and Ageing. 2016

75 Laukkanen T., Khan H., Zaccardi F., Laukkanen J. A. Association between sauna bathing and fatal cardiovascular and all-cause mortality events. JAMA Internal Medicine. 2015;175(4):542–548

76 Kihara T., Miyata M., Fukudome T., et al. Waon therapy improves the prognosis of patients with chronic heart failure. Journal of Cardiology. 2009;53(2):214–218.

77 Matsumoto S., Shimodozono M., Etoh S., Miyata R., Kawahira K. Effects of thermal therapy combining sauna therapy and underwater exercise in patients with fibromyalgia. Complementary Therapies in Clinical Practice. 2011;17(3):162–166.

78 Oosterveld F. G. J., Rasker J. J., Floors M., et al. Infrared sauna in patients with rheumatoid arthritis and ankylosing spondylitis. Clinical Rheumatology. 2009;28(1):29–34.

79 Katriina Kukkonen-Harjula & Kyllikki Kauppinen (2006) Health effects and risks of sauna bathing, International Journal of Circumpolar Health, 65:3, 195-205.

80 Joseph Charles Maroon, Jeffrey W. Bost, ω-3 Fatty acids (fish oil) as an anti-inflammatory: an alternative to nonsteroidal anti-inflammatory drugs for discogenic pain, Surgical Neurology, Volume 65, Issue 4, 2006, Pages 326-331.

81 Opperman M, Marais de W, Spinnler Benade AJ. Analysis of omega-3 fatty acid content of South African fish oil supplements. Cardiovasc J Afr. 2011;22(6):324–329. doi:10.5830/CVJA-2010-080.

82 https://www.bda.uk.com/foodfacts/omega3.pdf

83 Chris M. Bleakley & Gareth W. Davison (2010) Cryotherapy and inflammation: evidence beyond the cardinal signs, Physical Therapy Reviews, 15:6, 430-435.

84 Edzard Ernst, Veronika Fialka, Ice freezes pain? A review of the clinical effectiveness of analgesic cold therapy, Journal of Pain and Symptom Management, Volume 9, Issue 1, 1994, Pages 56-59.

85 Shephard RJ. Fat metabolism, exercise, and the cold. Canadian Journal of Sport Sciences. 1992. Jun;17(2):83-90.

86 Giemza, C., Matczak-Giemza, M., Ostrowska, B., Biec, E., Dolinski, M. (2014). Effect of cryotherapy on the lumbar spine in elderly men with back pain. Aging Male. 17(3). 183-188.

87 Nugraha, B., Gunther, J.T., Rawert, H., Siegert, R., Gutenbrunner, C. (2015) Effects of whole body cryo-chamber therapy on pain in patients with chronic low back pain: a prospective double blind randomised controlled trial. European Journal of Physical Rehabilitative Medicine. 51. 143-148.

88 Isabelle Aeberli, Philipp A Gerber, Michel Hochuli, Sibylle Kohler, Sarah R Haile, Ioanna Gouni-Berthold, Heiner K Berthold, Giatgen A Spinas, Kaspar Berneis, Low to moderate sugar-sweetened beverage consumption impairs glucose and lipid metabolism and promotes inflammation in healthy young men: a randomized controlled trial, The American Journal of Clinical Nutrition, Volume 94, Issue 2, August 2011, Pages 479–485.

89 K.G. Nevin, T. Rajamohan, Beneficial effects of virgin coconut oil on lipid parameters and in vitro LDL oxidation, Clinical Biochemistry, Volume 37, Issue 9, 2004, Pages 830-835.

90 Fabíola Lacerda Pires Soares, Rafael de Oliveira Matoso, Lílian Gonçalves Teixeira, Zélia Menezes, Solange Silveira Pereira, Andréa Catão Alves, Nathália Vieira Batista, Ana Maria Caetano de Faria, Denise Carmona Cara, Adaliene Versiani Matos Ferreira, Jacqueline Isaura Alvarez-Leite, Gluten-free diet reduces adiposity, inflammation and insulin resistance associated with the induction of PPAR-alpha and PPAR-gamma expression. The Journal of Nutritional Biochemistry, Volume 24, Issue 6, 2013, Pages 1105-1111.

91 Shaik-Dasthagirisaheb, Y.B. et al., 2013. Role of vitamins D, E and C in immunity and inflammation. *Journal of Biological Regulators and Homeostatic Agents.* **27**(2). 291-295.

92 Korntner, S., Kunkel, N., Lehner, C. et al. A high-glucose diet affects Achilles tendon healing in rats. Sci Rep 7, 780 (2017).

WELLBEING & THE POWER OF YOUR MIND

1 Brinjikji W, Luetmer PH, Comstock B, et al. Systematic literature review of imaging features of spinal degeneration in asymptomatic populations. AJNR Am J Neuroradiol. 2015;36(4):811–816.

2 Negendank, W.G., Fernandez–Madrid, F.R., Heilbrun, L.K. and Teitge, R.A. (1990), Magnetic resonance imaging of meniscal degeneration in asymptomatic knees. J. Orthop. Res., 8: 311-320.

3 Okada, E., Matsumoto, M., Fujiwara, H. et al. Disc degeneration of cervical spine on MRI in patients with lumbar disc herniation: comparison study with asymptomatic volunteers Eur Spine J (2011) 20: 585.

4 Puentedura, E.J., Leuw, A. (2012). A neuroscience approach to managing athletes with low back pain. Physical Therapy in Sport. 13. 123-133.

5 https://www.youtube.com/watch?v=gwd-wLdIHjs

6 Scott A. Hawkins, Stephen J. Hoch, Joan Meyers-Levy, Low-Involvement Learning: Repetition and Coherence in Familiarity and Belief, Journal of Consumer Psychology, Volume 11, Issue 1, 2001, Pages 1-11.

7 Majeed, M.H., Ali, A.A., Sudak, D.M. (2018). Mindfulness based interventions for chronic pain: evidence and application. Asian Journal of Psychiatry. 32. 79-82.

8 Tavallaei, V., Rezapour-Mirsaleh, Y., Rezaiemaram, P., Saadat, S.H. (2018). Mindfulness for female outpatients with chronic primary headaches: an internet-based bibliotherapy. Eur J Transl Myol. 28 (2): 175-184.

9 Stress, GCR, inflammation, and disease risk. Sheldon Cohen, Denise Janicki-Deverts, William J. Doyle, Gregory E. Miller, Ellen Frank, Bruce S. Rabin, Ronald B. Turner. Proceedings of the National Academy of Sciences Apr 2012, 109 (16) 5995-5999.

10 Alfred T Sapse, Stress, cortisol, interferon and "stress" diseases: I. Cortisol as the cause of "stress" diseases, Medical Hypotheses, Volume 13, Issue 1, 1984, Pages 31-44.

11 Alison N. Saul, Tatiana M. Oberyszyn, Christine Daugherty, Donna Kusewitt, Susie Jones, Scott Jewell, William B. Malarkey, Amy Lehman, Stanley Lemeshow, Firdaus S. Dhabhar, Chronic Stress and Susceptibility to Skin Cancer, *JNCI: Journal of the National Cancer Institute*, Volume 97, Issue 23, 7 December 2005, Pages 1760–1767.

12 Robles, T. F., Glaser, R., & Kiecolt-Glaser, J. K. (2005). Out of Balance: A New Look at Chronic Stress, Depression, and Immunity. *Current Directions in Psychological Science, 14*(2), 111–115.

13 M. Teut, E. J. Roesner, M. Ortiz, et al., "Mindful Walking in Psychologically Distressed Individuals: A Randomized Controlled Trial," Evidence-Based Complementary and Alternative Medicine, vol. 2013, Article ID 489856, 7 pages, 2013.

14 Putai Jin, Efficacy of Tai Chi, brisk walking, meditation, and reading in reducing mental and emotional stress, Journal of Psychosomatic Research, Volume 36, Issue 4, 1992, Pages 361-370.

15 Russell, D., Cutrona, C. E., Rose, J., & Yurko, K. (1984). Social and emotional loneliness: An examination of Weiss's typology of loneliness. *Journal of Personality and Social Psychology, 46*(6), 1313–1321.

16 Costigan M, Scholz J, Woolf CJ. Neuropathic pain: a maladaptive response of the nervous system to damage. Annu Rev Neurosci. 2009;32:1-32.

17 Goldstein P, Weissman-Fogel I, Shamay-Tsoory SG. The role of touch in regulating inter-partner physiological coupling during empathy for pain. Sci Rep. 2017 Jun 12;7(1):3252.

18 Ji RR, Nackley A, Huh Y, Terrando N, Maixner W. Neuroinflammation and Central Sensitization in Chronic and Widespread Pain. Anesthesiology. 2018 Aug;129(2): 343-366.

19 Birke H, Ekholm O, Højsted J, Sjøgren P, Kurita GP. Chronic Pain, Opioid Therapy, Sexual Desire, and Satisfaction in Sexual Life: A Population-Based Survey. Pain Med. 2019 Jun 1;20(6):1132-1140.

20 Matsuura T, Motojima Y, Kawasaki M, Ohnishi H, Sakai A, Ueta Y. Relationship Between Oxytocin and Pain Modulation and Inflammation. J UOEH. 2016;38(4):325-334.

21 Sidorkewicz N, McGill SM. Documenting female spine motion during coitus with a commentary on the implications for the low back pain patient. Eur Spine J. 2015 Mar; 24(3):513-20.

22 Sidorkewicz N, McGill SM. Male spine motion during coitus: implications for the low back pain patient. Spine (Phila Pa 1976). 2014 Sep 15;39(20):1633-9.

23 Stephens R, Atkins J, Kingston A. Swearing as a response to pain. Neuroreport. 2009 Aug 5;20(12):1056-60.

24 Stephens R, Umland C. Swearing as a response to pain-effect of daily swearing frequency. J Pain. 2011 Dec;12(12):1274-81.

25 Chen LF, Vander Weg MW, Hofmann DA, Reisinger HS. The Hawthorne Effect in Infection Prevention and Epidemiology. Infect Control Hosp Epidemiol. 2015 Dec; 36(12):1444-50.

26 Hanning U, Roesler A, Peters A, Berger K, Baune BT. Structural brain changes and all-cause mortality in the elderly population-the mediating role of inflammation. Age (Dordr). 2016 Dec;38(5-6):455-464.

27 https://www.who.int/news-room/fact-sheets/detail/mental-health-of-older-adults

28 Bernardo TC, Marques-Aleixo I, Beleza J, Oliveira PJ, Ascensão A, Magalhães J. Physical Exercise and Brain Mitochondrial Fitness: The Possible Role Against Alzheimer's Disease. Brain Pathol. 2016 Sep;26(5):648-63.

29 Khazaee-Pool M, Sadeghi R, Majlessi F, Rahimi Foroushani A. Effects of physical exercise programme on happiness among older people. J Psychiatr Ment Health Nurs. 2015 Feb;22(1):47-57.

30 Son WM, Sung KD, Cho JM, Park SY. Combined exercise reduces arterial stiffness, blood pressure, and blood markers for cardiovascular risk in postmenopausal women with hypertension. Menopause. 2017 Mar;24(3):262-268.

31 Kuiper JS, Zuidersma M, Oude Voshaar RC, Zuidema SU, van den Heuvel ER, Stolk RP, Smidt N. Social relationships and risk of dementia: A systematic review and meta-analysis of longitudinal cohort studies. Ageing Res Rev. 2015 Jul;22:39-57.

32 Zhong G, Wang Y, Zhang Y, Guo JJ, Zhao Y. Smoking is associated with an increased risk of dementia: a meta-analysis of prospective cohort studies with investigation of potential effect modifiers. PLoS One. 2015 Mar 12;10(3):e0118333.

33 http://www.exeter.ac.uk/news/featurednews/title_409094_en.html

34 Bang KS, Lee I, Kim S, Lim CS, Joh HK, Park BJ, Song MK. The Effects of a Campus Forest-Walking Program on Undergraduate and Graduate Students' Physical and Psychological Health. Int J Environ Res Public Health. 2017 Jul 5;14(7). pii: E728

35 Alquist J, Baumeister RF. Self-control: limited resources and extensive benefits. Wiley Interdiscip Rev Cogn Sci. 2012 May;3(3):419-423.